CW01375792

Resource Guide to Accompany

Breastfeeding and Human Lactation

Jan Riordan, Ed.D., ARNP, IBCLC, FAAN
Associated Professor of Nursing, Wichita State University
Research Consultant, St. Joseph Medical Center
Wichita, Kansas

Kathleen G. Auerbach, Ph.D., IBCLC
Complemental Faculty Member, Department of Maternal-Child Nursing
Rush-Presbyterian-St. Luke's Medical Center
Chicago, Illinois
Lactation Consultant and Researcher (Private Practice)
Homewood, Illinois

Jones and Bartlett Publishers
Sudbury, Massachusetts

Boston London Singapore

Editorial, Sales, and Customer Service Offices
Jones and Bartlett Publishers
40 Tall Pine Drive
Sudbury, MA 01776
(508) 443-5000
(800) 832-0034

Jones and Bartlett Publishers International
Barb House, Barb Mews
London W6 7PA
UK

Copyright © 1996 by Jones and Bartlett Publishers, Inc.

All rights reserved. No part of the material protected by this copyright notice may be reproduced or utilized in any form, electronic or mechanical, including photocopying, recording, or by any information storage and retrieval system, without written permission from the copyright owner.

ISBN 0-7637-0220-X

Printed in the United States of America
00 99 98 97 96 10 9 8 7 6 5 4 3 2 1

TABLE OF CONTENTS

INTRODUCTION

The *Resource Guide to Accompany Breastfeeding and Human Lactation*, an accompanying volume to *Breastfeeding and Human Lactation* and its *Study Guide,* is designed for educators to develop breastfeeding education programs and for lactation consultants who are looking for resources for their practice. Camera ready materials in this *Guide* will be helpful for deve-loping lectures, selecting topics for guest presentations, organizing discussions, suggesting student activities, and identifying appropriate audio-visual materials. Overhead transparency masters are provided to extend and expand on the materials in the primary text. Lactation consultants will find documents they need to use in clinical practice, such as forms for billing, insurance, assessment, consent, clinical care paths, and client instruction sheets.

Readers may duplicate certain pages without fear of copyright violation; for example, those meant for use as transparencies/overheads.

Each chapter contains:

• **An overview paragraph** describes the chapter contents in *Breastfeeding and Human Lactation*;

• **A definition and brief discussion of each of the Key Concepts** identified in the *Study Guide* for each chapter in the text.

• **Readings for Further Reference.** Supplementary publications important to understanding a particular topic add detail to each key concept or topic.

In planning lecture material and student activities, the instructor is urged to first go to the references noted in the text for detail pertaining to each key concept or question topic. Additional readings speci-fic to certain suggested activities are also offered in this Resource Guide.

• **Learning Activities.** Either an Instructor's Activity (I) or a Student Activity (S). Each suggests additional instructor lecture information, classroom discussion, or student activities that extend the information in the text. Items can be used as the foci for student assignments, such as paper topics, or discussions in class. In some cases, several different projects or assignments are offered for the same topic. This provides alternatives that take into account student skills and orientations and whether the student is at a beginning or advanced stage of learning.

• **Student Projects that Require Data Gathering.** Those activities requiring that students survey or interview breastfeeding mothers or other persons can be found in this special section.

• **Audio-visual materials.** Slides, videos, audio tapes and other AV's that reinforce learning are listed in a special Appendix and keyed to specific chapters where their use is recommended.

• **Educational Course Offerings.** To assist students seeking additional programs, see the listing of those institutions offering study opportunities that provide a minimum of 15 contact hours of lactation study as of the date of publication.

• **Transparency/Overhead Masters.** Copy-ready transparency masters may be used to assist the instructor in presenting material for detailed exposition or class discussion. Students may also use these masters to illustrate key points of assignments.

• **Appendices.** Some forms or other documents and breastfeeding educational materials can be found in this section. These items can be freely copied and are so identified. Others are provided with ordering information from the original copyright holder

CHAPTER 1

Tides in Breastfeeding Practice

This chapter focuses on the many ways in which breastfeeding has been practiced over time. After reading this chapter, the reader will have a deeper understanding of the ways in which breastfeeding reflects, and is governed by, cultural, social, and environmental conditions. Such forces are not an issue only in contemporary society, but have structured how, when, why, and in what situations breastfeeding is encouraged, accepted, or proscribed.

KEY CONCEPTS

1. **Breastfeeding Practices** - Those customs or beliefs and/or activities that serve to structure how, when, where, and by whom breastfeeding occurs. Each culture maintains its own beliefs about breastfeeding; each culture defines when it is considered most–or least–appropriate. In all cultures, dysjunctions between some beliefs and some practices may co-exist. This is more likely when change, both social and technological, is rapid.

2. **Breastfeeding Promotion** - Those actions, written promulgations, and oral statements, which individually and collectively, result in advertising, publicity, advocacy, and/or endorsement of breastfeeding. Such promotion may be accomplished by an individual, by small or large groups, by lay or professional organizations, or by government agencies speaking for the nation or one or more national leaders.

3. **Breastfeeding Regulation** - The control of breastfeeding as an activity or action through the structuring of specific practices, such as requiring that it occur at specified intervals, or for particular periods of time, or in identified "appropriate" places, and the like.

4. **Hand-feeding** - The term applied to artificial feeding of foods or fluids other than human milk; the term probably derives from identification of the first vessel other than the breast used to hold such foods. The term is now used to refer to a wide variety of containers, including animal horns, pottery, metal, plastic, and glass, the most recent version of which is the feeding bottle topped with a rubberized teat set. Regardless of the contents or type of vessel used, each of the alternatives to breastfeeding harbors risks that do not exist when the baby feeds directly from her or his mother's breasts.

5. **Infant Mortality** - The number of infants who die prior to their first birthday anniversary. Often, infant mortality is expressed as a rate; that is, the number of death per 1,000 or 100,000 or 1 million live births. The infant mortality rate is often used as a measure of the health status of a society.

6. **Manufactured baby milks** - Any fluid given to a baby as a substitute, replacement, or complement–partially or completely–for human milk, and prepared for commercial sale and distribution.

7. **Mixed feeds** - Any feed of mashed, semi-solid, or solid food given to an infant in addition to fluid nutriment. In some societies, such mixed feeds are introduced shortly after birth; in other societies, their introduction and use represents a later developmental milestone.

8. **Pre-lacteal feeds** - Feeds given to a neonate in advance of his/her first feeding from the breast. Such feeds may be liquid, pre-masticated, or semi-solid mashed food and may vary by culture, as will the rationale supporting the practice.

9. **Wet-Nursing** - One alternative to breastfeeding by the infant's own mother; often resulting in payment (monetary or in kind) to the lactating woman who is suckling the infant. In periods when wet-nursing was an accepted practice, the woman who served in this capacity was often accorded an honored position in the household. In modern societies, the practice is less appreciated and less visible. Where it is practiced, often the mother and the wet-nursing individual are related to one another; i.e., sisters.

10. **WHO Code** - A code designed to govern the marketing of artificial baby milks. It is neither a code of ethics nor a regulation, the violation of which results in a fine or other punitive action. Individual nations worldwide have adopted the original Code, or modified it in ways specific to their country. In 1994, the United States, previously the sole negative vote when first ratified in 1981, ratified the WHO Code.

11. **WIC Program** - A supplemental food program in the United States for women with low incomes, defined as a percentage per family size of the federally-determined poverty level. In most cases, artificial baby milk is offered through this program as well as additional foods for women and children through their fifth birthday anniversary. The giving of artificial milks by this program has been implicated in low breastfeeding rates by participants. However, since 1988, breastfeeding has been actively promoted by the WIC program, with varying success. Although federally funded, individual states administer WIC funds.

READINGS FOR FURTHER REFERENCE

Armstrong, HC, and Sokol, E: *The International Code of Marketing of Breast-Milk Substitutes: What It Means for Mothers and Babies World-wide*.. Evanston, IL: International Lactation Consultant Association, 1994 (Order from ILCA Office, 200 N. Michigan Avenue, Suite 300, Chicago, IL 60601 USA)

Auerbach, KG: Breastfeeding promotion: why it doesn't work (editorial). *J Hum Lact* 6:46-48,1990.

Fildes, V: *Breasts, Bottles and Babies,* Edinburgh: Edinburgh University Press, 1986.

Palmer, G: *The Politics of Breastfeeding*. London: Pandora Press, 1988.

Tamagond B, K, S: Effect on neonatal feeding practices of a program to promote colostrum feeding in India. *J Nutr Educ* 24:29-32, 1992.

Valaitis, RK, Shea, E: An evaluation of breastfeeding promotion literature: does it really promote breastfeeding? *Can J Public Health* 84: 24-27, 1993.

Van Esterik, P: *Beyond the Breast-Bottle Controversy*. New Brunswick, NJ: Rutgers University Press, 1989.

Winikoff,B, Castle, MA, Laukaran, VH, Eds: *Feeding Infants in Four Societies: Causes and Consequences of Mothers' Choices.* NY: Greenwood Press, 1988.

LEARNING ACTIVITIES

1. Which breastfeeding practices appear to have existed in one or more cultures for more than two hundred years? Develop a chart that traces a particular belief over time and across cultures. (See Van Esterik) (I)

2. Review TR 1-1 and 1-2. (I)
   a. To what audience(s) is each of these slogans about breastfeeding aimed?
   b. What additional slogans might you suggest? What is their intended audience?

3. Examine the rationale discussed in the editorial by Auerbach and illustrated in TR 1-3. (I)
   a. Ask your students to discuss the relationship between promotion, support, and protection, as identified in the above editorial?
   b. Are the distinctions clear?
   c. Are they appropriate?
   d. What advantages/disadvantages do you see in using the analogy of the three-legged stool?
   e. What other analogy than a three-legged stool might be more illustrative of the problem?

4. Ask your students to identify at least three different examples of breastfeeding promotion that they encounter in their everyday lives; three examples of breastfeeding support; three examples of protection of breastfeeding. (S)
   a. Also list at least three examples of each of the following:
      1) bottle-feeding promotion
      2) bottle-feeding protection
      3) bottle-feeding support
   b. What does the above exercise say about the society with which these students are most familiar?

5. Ask the students to review the role of the breastfeeding advocate as identified in text Chapter 3, pp. 69-74. Then ask them to devise a plan that advocates breastfeeding in a setting which previously has not resulted in a high rate of breastfeeding initiation or extended past one year duration. (S)

6. Ask the students to (S):
   a. prepare a newspaper or magazine advertisement using fewer than 50 words, whose aim is to promote breastfeeding. Ask them to write such ad copy for at least three of the following audiences:
      1) a group of Rotary Club members, 80% of whom are men in their 50's
      2) low-income families residing in an urban high rise complex
      3) farm families whose contacts with non-relatives is infrequent but intense when they do occur;
      4) a local chapter of the American Association of Businesswomen;
      5) a group of recent Asian immigrants, who believe that the country in which they now live is a bottle-feeding society;
      6) migrant farm workers who are semi- to illiterate in the dominant language;
      7) daycare workers, most of whose clientele have infants younger than 1 year of age;
      8) the readership of a large metropolitan daily newspaper;
      9) a group of pregnant women who will see the completed promotional piece in their doctor's office;
      10) physicians in a developing country (pick the country first)
      11) physicians in a developed country (pick the country first)
      12) midwives/nurses in a developing country (pick the country first)
      13) midwives/nurses in a developed country (pick the country first)

7. Ask your students to review Valaitis and Shea. (S)
   a. Have them select at least six different brochures/pamphlets about breastfeeding that they obtain from a local physician's office, prenatal clinic, health department, or other source.
   b. Ask them to conduct a content analysis similar to the one reported by Valaitis. How are their findings similar to/different from that of Valaitis and Shea?
   c. Their report of their findings can then presented as a paper. Brief summaries can be part of a classroom discussion.

8. How is breastfeeding regulated in your local community? How do you know such regulation exists? (I)

9. What are at least two risks of each of the following examples of hand-feeding? (I)
   a. Container
      1) animal horn
      2) metal cup or bowl
      3) pottery or glass cup or bowl
      4) plastic or glass bottle
      5) rubber(ized) teat set
   b. Fluid or food
      1) animal milks
      2) manufactured baby milk
      3) semi-solid food
      4) human milk

10. Explain why the agricultural revolution contributed to the rise in artificial hand-feeding. (See Palmer; esp. Chapter 5) (I)

11. Trace the development of alternative baby milks from individualized formulae to mass-produced brands with standardized identified ingredients. (I)

12. Discuss the risks of each method of hand-feeding, focusing on both the container and what it contains. How might these risks be reduced? For each identified way to reduce the risk of hand-feeding, ask the students: is this risk reduction method available world-wide? Does it represent other costs? If so, which one(s)? (I)

13. Name at least seven brands of manufactured baby milk. Which brands are most prevalent in the local commu- nity? Where are the others distributed? (I)

14. Send students to three different grocery stores or other commercial outlets for manufactured baby milk. In addition to their own questions, ask them to describe: (S)
   a. How are the baby milks displayed?
   b. For each brand, what is the cost (comparing same size containers and types of baby milk)
   c. How much will this be for 1 month, 6 months, 1 year?
   d. Ask the store manager how often/when such items go "on sale." If not a sale item, why is it not handled in this manner?
   e. What brand and type of industrial milk is the "best" seller? How does the manager track such sales? How long has this been true? If differences in "best sellers" have occurred, what accounts for this change?
   f. What feeding or equipment items for breastfeeding mothers are found in this store? Where are they displayed (relative to placement of the commercial baby milks)?

15. Ask your students to conduct a content analysis of advertisements for: (S)
   a. manufactured milks
   b. feeding bottles/cups
   c. teats/rubber nipple sets
   d. infant foods (semi-solid)
   e. pacifiers, teething rings, etc.
   f. other baby items
   Specifically:
      1) Where are such ads found?
      2) What is their intended audience?
      3) What is the suggested infant age for use of such items?
      4) What is the cost of such items?

16. How might the 1895 advertisement (p. 9 in text) be used as an inducement for mothers to artificially feed their babies? How does this ad differ from (and how is it similar to) current advertisements seen in magazines for women? Where are most ads for artificial milks found today? Why? (I)

17. Define wet nursing. How is it related to the practice of cross-nursing in the United States? Identify at least three factors that contributed to the decline of wet nursing on the European continent in the 19th century. What three concerns might limit the practice of cross-nursing today? (I)

18. Review the practice of wet nursing in a society of your choosing prior to the 19th century. (See Fildes: *Breasts, Bottles and Babies,* esp. Chapters 5-7) Also review the practice in a contemporary society. Point out for your students the differences and similarities in beliefs about wet-nursing in these two settings at different times. (I)

19. Refer to TR 1-5 and 1- 6. Begin your discussion by asking your students why each element in the WHO Code summary is important in developing countries, developed countries. Then ask your students to read the Anderson/Sokol monograph pertaining to the Summary Elements of the WHO Code. After reading this material, ask them to propose two practice recommendations for each element in the Code. (S)

20. Review two separate countries' experiences with the WHO Code. One nation should be considered a developing country and one a developed country. Compare and contrast their involvement with the WHO Code. How have their respective activities pertaining to the WHO Code elements related to maternal breastfeeding experiences in that country? (I)

21. Ask your students to assume that they have just been appointed Federal Secretary/ Minister of Health for Infants or Young Children. The national leadership has concluded that the WHO Code should be completely implemented in your country. The job of the student, as policy leader, is to determine a) how, b) when, c) where, d) why the WHO Code is to be implemented. The student's paper—or oral presentation—shall address each of the above four issues. Encourage creativity. (S)

22. Ask your students to visit three different WIC offices and to describe what they have observed; specifically... (S)
    a. how is breastfeeding advertised/encouraged?
    b. how is artificial milk use encouraged/advertised?
    c. what is the breastfeeding rate of the infants who participate in the program? How do the workers/administrative personnel track this rate?
    d. what changes have occurred in breastfeeding promotion and assistance in the WIC office in the past five years? What stimulated these changes and what has resulted?

24. If your country is not the US, describe a program, if such exists, that provides assistance to low income women. In what ways(s) is this program similar to the US WIC program? In what way(s) does it differ? (I)

25. You are asked to discuss*/design a program of breastfeeding promotion and assistance for women with the following characteristics: (S)
    a. low income
    b. a recent immigrant to the country
    c. member of a minority ethnic/racial group
    d. unmarried
    e. under age 19

    *Undergraduate students will discuss in class; graduate students will design a program.

26. Ask the students to explain the importance of the graphic in TR 1-4. (S)
    a. What is its meaning for mothers and babies?
    b. What is its significance in the students' culture, the health care system with which the students are most familiar?

CHAPTER 2

The Cultural Context of Breastfeeding

The study of culture begins with examining one's own cultural values and then those of other cultural groups. The seeds of a culture are planted through the patterns of childbearing and childrearing practices. Every culture has a dominant belief system that overlaps with folk health beliefs. Systematically assessing breastfeeding in a given culture includes gathering information on customs, values, communication, kinship patterns, health practices, religion, political systems and infant care and feeding practices.

KEY CONCEPTS

1. **Allopathic Medicine** - Dominant methods of medical care in Western societies; so-called "professional" medical care. Allopathic medicine, as defined in North American countries, is practiced in hospitals, medical offices, and community health departments.

2. **Childbirth** - Childbirth practices, like breastfeeding practices, are affected by culture. Since both breastfeeding and childbearing are intertwined, it is essential to be informed on childbirth practices within a given culture if one is to understand breastfeeding practices.

3. **Colostrum** - Many cultures regard colostrum as a harmful substance. This is an example of a breastfeeding practice that should be changed, since it robs the neonate of vital immunological and nutritional components.

4. **Cultural relativism** - Recognition and appreciation of cultural differences. Approaching each breastfeeding client with respect and deference to her cultural background.

5. **Ethnocentrism** - Judging the world by one's own standards, or believing that one's own group values are the only acceptable values. Viewing the world where oneself is the center.

6. **Food restrictions** - Food restrictions during lactation are common practices and vary according to the culture. Generally, cultural food restrictions are similar to those for sick people within a particular culture.

7. **Galactogogues** - Foods that are believed to increase the supply of breastfmilk and vary according to the culture.

8. **Infant care** - Swaddling, sleeping together, special clothing, and ways of carrying of baby are all influenced by cultural values and mores.

9. **Language** - A systematic means of communicating ideas or feelings by the use of conventionalized signs, sounds, gestures or marks having understood meanings. Counseling breastfeeding women from diverse cultures requires special skills and assistance.

10. **Maternal foods** - Despite the wide diversity of cultural foods consumed by breastfeeding women throughout the planet, breastmilk is amazingly homogenous.

11. **Rituals** - A special behavior heavily influenced by culture that may affect breastfeeding either positively or negatively. For example, routine separation and mother following birth is a negative ritual.

12. **Vegetarianism** - Avoiding meat in the diet is entirely compatible with lactation if the mother consumes adequate protein and vitamin B_{12}.

13. **Weaning** - a process during which mothers introduce their infant to culturally assigned foods. Weaning begins with the introduction of sources of food other than breastmilk and ends with the last feeding at the breast. Weaning may be gradual, deliberate, or abrupt.

14. **Wet nursing** - Breastfeeding a child that was birthed by another woman, a long-established traditional practice.

READINGS FOR FURTHER REFERENCE

Maher, V, Ed: *The Anthropology of Breast-Feeding: Natural Law or Social Construct.* Oxford, UK: Berg Publishers Limited, 1992.

Raphael, D: *The Tender gift: Breastfeeding.* New York, Schocken Books; 1976, see esp. Chapter 11.

Riordan, J: *A Practical Guide to Breastfeeding.* St. Louis: C.V. Mosby Company, 1983; see esp. Chapters 14-18.

Stuart-Macadam, P, Dettwyer, KA, Eds: *Breastfeeding: Biocultural Perspectives.* New York: Aldine de Gruyter, 1995; see esp. Chapters 2-5, 7 and 8.

Van Esterik, P: *Beyond the Breast-Bottle Controversy.* New Brunswick, NJ: Rutgers University Press, 1989.

LEARNING ACTIVITIES

1. Identify the different cultures mentioned in Chapter 1. For each culture: (I)
   a. Discuss at least one practice related to breastfeeding.
   b. Ask the students to identify whether a particular breastfeeding practice has positive value, negative value, or is neutral as it relates to current knowledge about breastfeeding. [This question cannot be completely answered without also referring to some of the information found in Chapter 9.)

2. Define allopathic medicine and contrast it with folk/traditional medicine. (I,S)

3. Invite four mothers to class, two of whom have given birth at home, and two of whom have given birth in a hospital setting. Ask each mother to describe why she chose the birth site she did, and whether she would use the same setting for a future birth. Under what circumstances would she choose another site, and what site would that be? (I)

4. What is colostrum? Describe ways of identifying colostrum in human milk samples and the significance for a new mother of colostrum in her milk. (I,S)

5. Define ethnocentrism and contrast it with cultural relativism. (I, S)

6. Discuss how the timing and use of mixed feeds... (I)
   a. varies by culture/society (See Winikoff, Castle and Laukaran; Chapter 1)
   b. may symbolize becoming 'human' or a progression from infancy to early childhood
   c. the risks of replacing human milk feeds with mixed feeds prior to infant readiness
   d. the relationship of use of such feeds to infant physiology, such as the extrusion reflex.

7. Identify at least three different examples of pre-lacteal feeds in the local community. Why are they given? If they are <u>not</u> used, why are they not part of the neonate's early life experience? (I)

8. Review how prelacteal feeds are related to different belief systems pertaining to human milk, early milk (colostrum), later milk and how educating mothers regarding the value of colostrum may change early breastfeeding behavior. (See Tamagond B and K S, Chapter 1) (I)

9. Assign students to interview people from other countries about childbirth and infant feeding practices in their culture of origin. Structure the interview using the Guide of Assessing Culture in Chapter 2 (p. 31) (See TR 2-1). Compile the results of these interviews on a large sheet or on the blackboard. Have the class compare cross-cultural similarities and differences of childbearing and childrearing practices among difference cultures and regions of the world. (I)

10. Examine how different religious beliefs influence infant feeding patterns. (S)

11. Define vegetarianism and explain in what way(s) such a pattern of eating might influence a woman during her pregnancy, childbirth, and breastfeeding course. (I,S)

12. Distinguish between mother-determined and child-led weaning. When is each likely to occur? In what way(s) are different methods of weaning likely to influence mothers and their children? (I,S)

13. What is wet-nursing? How was it practiced in previous periods? currently? (I,S)

14. Review TR 2-2. Discuss each type of weaning. Ask the students to provide an example of each type of weaning and how cultures can influence weaning patterns and their timing of occurrence. (I, S)

CHAPTER 3

Families

This chapter focuses on the family as the small group in which breastfeeding takes place. How families evolve, the different forms they take over time, the effect of a baby on the family, the special needs of families of teen parents and low-income families—all are discussed in light of how this might affect the decision to breastfeed as well as how it is promoted.

KEY CONCEPTS

1. **Affiliation** - A sense by each family member that their connection with and to other family members differs from their connections with non-family individuals; a "we" vs. "they" notion, or a sense of "in-group" vs. "out-group" membership.

2. **Attachment** - Behavior that illustrates the unique connection between a mother or father and her/his child. Attachment may also accrue to other relationships, including those with extended family members, fictive kin, and other non-related (by blood or marriage) persons; however, in most societies strongest attachment ties are recognized between mother and/or father and child.

3. **Contracting stage** - The time in the family life cycle when its size is diminishing as one or more child members disperse elsewhere—to establish their own family of procreation, to establish a single adult household, or some other family form separate from their family of orientation.

4. **Couple stage** - That time in the family life cycle when its members include only a wife and a husband.

5. **Expanding stage** - That time in the family life cycle when new members are being added (usually by birth or adoption).

6. **Extended family** - A recognized group of related kin (by blood or marriage) which expands laterally as well as generationally from the nucleus of parents and children. Thus, grandparents and cousins, aunts and uncles are identified as part of a larger family group. In some cases, one or more of these extended kin may live in the same household.

7. **Family development theory** - A theoretical construct that seeks to identify key tasks occurring at specific periods in the "family life cycle." These tasks are thought to identify individual family members' roles and their relationships to other members of the family and to the group itself.

8. **Family of orientation** - The small group into which a child is born or adopted and usually raised to adulthood.

9. **Family of procreation** - The small group into which one marries, and bears and rears children. In some cases, a family of procreation may include no children, by choice or circumstance.

10. **Family functioning** - The degree to which a family, regardless of its stage, is fulfilling the needs of all its members and meeting of its group needs of self-care.

11. **Innovation-decision process** - One model designed to explain why some women choose to breastfeed while others do not.

12. **Nuclear family** - A small group whose members are related by blood or marriage that usually includes a male and a female parent and their biological and/ or adopted children.

READINGS FOR FURTHER REFERENCE

Friedman, MM: *Family Nursing: Theory and Practice*, 3rd ed. Norwalk, CT: Appleton and Eagle, 1992.

LEARNING ACTIVITIES

1. Ask your students to identify at least two examples of how family members distinguish themselves from other persons who are not identified as "family." (S)

2. Review the use of surnames. In what way(s) might the use of some surnames, but not others, be helpful in establishing connections between certain persons. How might such surname use illustrate keys to under standing male or female dominance? (I)

3. Your students are introduced to each of the following mothers: (S)
   a. Mary Lawson-Smith; her baby's surname is Lawson, the mother's original surname.
   b. Janice Jones; the baby's surname is Smith, the father's surname. (The father does not live with the mother or her child.)
   c. Katrina Williamson, who is married to John Williamson. Their baby's name is Williamson.
   What do each of these names suggest about family relationships?

4. Review how different routines that often occur in hospital can affect early post-birth attachment behaviors by focusing on the following: (I)
   a. labor anesthesia
   b. episiotomies
   c. early separation of mother and neonate
   d. restricted visiting patterns by other family members
   e. duration of hospital stay
   f. sleeping arrangements of mother and baby

5. Ask the students to... (S)
   a. identify ways in which paternal attachment is similar to maternal attachment;
   b. ways in which paternal attachment differs from maternal attachment;
   c. ways in which cultural beliefs affect attachment behavior.

6. Describe how sibling attachments are developed and how they alter parent-child relationshiips within the same family. Refer to TR 3-3. Then compare TR 3-3 with TR 3-1 and 3-2. (I)

7. Ask the students to observe a mother-to-mother support group and to identify attachment behaviors seen there. Ask them to note how mothers in the group describe paternal attachment behavior. (S)

8. Discuss each of the nine reasons for having a baby listed in Chapter 3. In each case, discuss the... (I)
   a. positive effects of maternal and paternal attachment to an infant
   b. negative effects of maternal and paternal attachment to an infant on the parents whose reason for having the baby is specific to one of each of those nine options.

9. Ask the students to examine the contracting stage in each of the following families: (S)
   a. four-person family of two adults and two children
   b. three-person family with one child
   c. eight-person single-parent family
   d. six-person family whose four children range from a newborn to a 22-year old recent college graduate
   e. four-person three-generation family of one child, one parent and two elderly grandparents
   In each case, ask the students to consider...
   a. the effect of one child's leave-taking on that same child*

b. the effect of one child's leave-taking on other siblings (if any)
c. the effect of the child's leave-taking on the parent(s)
d. the effect of the child's leave-taking on the grandparent(s), if any
*in situations with more than one child, the student may select who is the index child

10. Examine how a family in the contracting stage (one or more children are leaving) might be affected by, and in turn affect, the mother's breastfeeding experience with a new infant. (I)

11. Ask the students to examine each of the tasks identified by Duvall (pp. 56-57 in the text). For each task, the students will discuss... (S)
    a. *why* the task is important to later family roles and responsibilities
    b. *how* the task can be accomplished
    c. *the separate roles* of each marital partner in completing the task
    d. how *failure to complete the task* will influence related tasks at later stages
    e. different *ways* in which cultural/ethnic/racial identity might influence each task

12. Ask the students to discuss how... (S)
    a. a short couple stage (through birth of the first child) can influence later family functioning
    b. elongation of the couple stage (through delay of the birth of the first child) can influence later family functioning

13. How, when, and for how long families add members will influence the family life cycle for decades. Compare and discuss the following family situations: (I)
    a. family whose two children are 11 months apart
    b. family whose three children are 1 year, 6 years, and 12 years old, respectively
    c. family whose five children are newborn, 2 years, 3 1/2 years, 5 years, and 7 years old, respectively
    d. family with six children whose youngest is 2 years old and whose oldest child is 19 years old [students select ages of 'in-between' children]

    For each family, ask the students to identify stage-specific tasks the family is engaging in *now* (**NB:** Some tasks from different stages may be relevant simultaneously). In addition, (S)
    a. For each family, for how long is the expanding stage experienced? How might this influence the duration of later family stages?
    b. How will simultaneously engaged tasks from different stages influence each family's functioning?
    c. How might the age of the oldest child predict tasks that are specific to the younger child(ren)?
    d. Which family theory is easiest to use in discussing a particular family's stage-specific tasks? why?
    e. Which family theory represents the greatest complexity of combinations of stage-specific tasks? How might the family researcher resolve such complexity into a coherent understanding of each family's tasks?
    f. The above questions may form the basis for a panel discussion, a paper, or an oral presentation.

14. Ask the students to trace their own family tree through at least three generations vertically, and as many laterally-related individuals as they can identify. In each case, they should... (S)
    a. identify how each related individual is named; i.e., the relationship to the index person (her/himself), and whether that named relationship is referred to when addressing that individual, such as Aunt Mary or Grandfather George/Smith.
    b. identify the age difference between the index person and each related individual. How does this age difference govern the kin relationship?
    c. Are any of these relationships considered closer than others? more distant? What elements contribute to the degree of closeness/distance felt? What does this reveal about the nature of extended kin relationships in this student's life and culture?
    d. How many extended kin relationships (exclusive of siblings and parents) can the student identify? How is this family connected to the larger world, and what does it mean for the student's sense of family?

15. Ask the students to write a paper identifying the five universals considered to apply to any group called a family in terms of their own extended family. (S)

16. Review how Duvall and Aldous differ from one another in their explication of family development theory. In this review, compare their view with the simplest four-stage view of family life (couple, expansion, stable, contracting) and the family members' relative responsibilities. (I)

17. Divide the students into groups. For each group, assign a particular family stage which they represent. Ask them to identify five problems "their" family life cycle stage may experience and, for each, how those problems can be resolved. (S)

18. Ask the students to identify their family of orientation. (S)
    a. In what way(s) does it differ from the "ideal theoretical" family of two parents and four children, two of whom are female and two of whom are male?
    b. Using TR-13 as a guide, what relationships are represented by that particular family of orientation?
    c. What relationships are missing and how has this influenced the remaining family members?

19. Ask the students to identify their family of procreation. (S)
    a. If they have not yet entered into such a family, ask them to use another family with which they are familiar <u>other</u> than their parent(s)' family of procreation. This exercise could form the basis for a term paper.
    b. In what stage is their family of procreation?
    c. How might the addition of.... affect their family of procreation?
        1) one child in 10 months
        2) two children over the next 5 years
        3) one planned birth
        4) one planned birth and one unplanned birth of twins
        5) two unplanned births within 18 months
        6) awareness of inability to have (any more) children
    d. How might the moving into the household of.... affect their family of procreation?
        1) an aged mother (in-law)
        2) an aged father (in-law)
        3) a pair of aged relatives
        4) a distant relation without other identified family to turn to whose terminal illness has recently been identifed as AIDS.
        5) a lateral relative (aunt/uncle/cousin) who has been homeless for two years prior to his/her arrival on your doorstep after many years of minimal communication
        6) a much-loved eccentric relative you haven't seen for many years

20. Review the Innovation Decision-Making Process (see TR 3-4). For each step, define what is meant and give an example for each of the following women: (I)
    a. a low-income woman
    b. a young career professional who is newly pregnant
    c. a middle-class woman living in a suburban area
    d. a single woman who is raising two children
    e. an immigrant whose language skills are improving, but are not yet sufficient to enable her to get a job

21. Review some of the frequently-mentioned obstacles to breastfeeding among low-income families, including the following: (I)
    a. mother's age
    b. ethnic/racial group identification
    c. lack of support for breastfeeding
    d. lack of information
    e. hospital routines
    f. baby milk marketing practices
    g. timing of solid food introduction
    h. social support

i. acceptance of breastfeeding as a maternal-child behavior
j. degree of breastfeeding promotion in the community
k. advocacy for breastfeeding in the community
For each of the above elements, ask the students to present examples where the element resulted in shorter duration of, or no, breastfeeding; more, or longer, breastfeeding. With each comparison, highlight what changed a negative outcome to a positive one.

22. Ask the students to write a paper explaining how they would affect a change toward greater initiation or longer duration of breastfeeding when one of the elements listed in Assignment #21 above currently has resulted in fewer women breastfeeding or in shorter duration of breastfeeding. In each paper, the student should review research studies supportive of their plan. (S)

23. Ask the students to explain why teenage mothers in the US and other developed countries are *less* likely to breastfeed than are older mothers. Their explanation should be based on interviews with at least 5 mothers aged 14-19 years old. (S)

24. Using a panel of women with one, two, three, four, or five or more children, ask each to tell the students about their infant feeding decisions (for each child) and why they made such a decision. After this presentation, ask the students to summarize those elements that contributed to the women's infant feeding decisions. What similarities do they discover? What differences are evident? (I/S)

25. Ask the students to identify their own nuclear family. What are its particular strengths? weaknesses? How does it differ from an extended family? (S)

26. Show your students TR 1-4. Explain how mother and baby are influenced first by one another and then, both individually and collectively by those persons, beliefs, and support mechanisms making up the local and broader societal contexts in which each mother and baby are found. (I)

CHAPTER 4

Anatomic and Biologic Imperatives

Breastfeeding involves anatomy and physiologic mechanisms of both the mother and infant in a symbiotic interchange. The mother's mammary development, breast and nipple structure and hormonal changes influence lactogenesis. The infant's oral development and suckling patterns equally influence breastfeeding. Early breastfeeding assessment is vital as it may detect solvable problems that may interfere with breastfeeding.

KEY CONCEPTS

Breast assessment - Both inspection and palpation are necessary for assessing the breast and nipples. Ideally it is done prenatally. Size, symmetry, and skin of the breasts are inspected for any deviations. Nipple function is assessed by palpation of the nipple.

Breast structure - The breast structure consists of highly vascular glandular and fibrous tissue. The basic unit for milk production is the *alveolus* which is surrounded by *myoepithelial cells* that eject milk into *ductules*. Each ductule merges into *lactiferous* or *mammary ducts* which empty into the *ampullae* or *lactiferous sinuses* behind the nipple. The major source for breast sensation is the fourth intercostal nerve.

Glactorrhea - Abnormal production of milk that may occur under psychological influences or be sign of a pituitary tumor.

Hormones - Prolactin and oxytocin are the major hormones that influence lactation. Prolactin is the principal hormone for milk biosynthesis. Oxytocin, secreted from the posterior pituitary is released during suckling and causes ejection of milk as well as uterine contractions.

Human placental lactogen (HPL) - Synthesized by the placenta and secreted in maternal serum during pregnancy. Its role in lactogenesis is not yet clear.

Insulin-like growth factor - An insulin-like factor in human milk thought to promote growth.

Lactogenesis - Milk synthesis and secretion. Initiation of milk synthesis postpartum is hormonally driven; continuation of milk production is driven by the frequency and quality of milk removal from the breasts. Lactogenesis is regulated through a feedback control system.

Mammary development - Breast development begins in fetal life and reaches maturation during pregnancy and lactation. At puberty, estrogen stimulates glandular growth, augmented by progesterone during ovulatory phases.

Newborn oral development - The oral and facial structure of the newborn and infant is configured to assist the newborn in holding the breast and removing milk during suckling. As the child grows, both soft and hard structures slowly change in structure and function to accommodate the introduction of solids. Rooting, suckling, and swallowing is established by 32 weeks gestation; smooth coordinated suckling, swallowing and breathing occurs later.

Pregnancy - Estrogen and progesterone stimulate ductal and lobe proliferation, and secretory activity. Colostrum is present during the second half of pregnancy.

Prolactin receptor theory - A biologic construct that proposes that the controlling factor of breastmilk output is the number of prolactin receptors rather than the amount of prolactin in the mother's serum.

Prolactin inhabiting factor (PIF) - A dopamine-like hypothalamic substance that inhibits prolactin. When PIF is suppressed, for example, by suckling breast pumping, prolactin levels rise.

Suckling/sucking - Terms used interchangeably to describe infant feeding at the breast. The use of one term over another has generated heated debate in the breastfeeding community.

Thyroid-stimulating hormone (TSH) - Thyroid hormones that promote mammary growth and lactogenesis.

Thyrotropin-releasing hormone (TRH) - Thought to increase TSH and prolactin levels. Its exact function is not yet clear.

READINGS FOR FUTHER REFERENCE

Lawrence, R: *Breastfeeding: A Guide for the Medical Profession*, 4th ed. St. Louis: C.V. Mosby, 1994; see esp. Chapters 2 and 3.

Mepham, TB: *Physiology of Lactation.* Philadelphia: Open University Press, 1987.

Neville, MC, Neifert, MR, Eds: *Lactation: Physiology, Nutrition, and Breast-Feeding.* New York: Plenum Press, 1983; see esp. Chapters 2-8.

LEARNING ACTIVITIES

1. To demonstrate flat vs. inverted vs. extended nipples, manual expression and correct finger placement during breastfeeding, use an almost-inflated ballon which has a "nipple" and darkened "areola." Overinflate a balloon to simulate engorgement; release air to simulate milk expression (and refer to TR 4-1). (I)

2. Use a model of the breast to demonstrating the flexibility of the nipple, nipple eversion, nipple inversion (refer to TR4-6 and 4-7). (I)

3. Invite a panel of four lactation consultants to class and ask each to outline how they assess the maternal breast and the breastfeeding encounter. (I)

4. Describe and define galactorrhea. Explain when it is likely to occur, under what circumstances, and when it can be considered an indicator of a problem. (I,S)

5. What are glucocorticoids? (I,S)

6. Review the different hormones that influence the lactation course (Refer to TR 4-2,4-3,4-4, and 4-5). (I,S)

7. Review the process of lactogenesis. Outline how you would explain the process to a woman who is unfamiliar with the physiology of breastfeeding. (S)

8. Distinguish between suckling and sucking. In what way is such a distinction important, irrelevant? (I,S)

9. Refer to TR 4-4 and 4-5. Develop a chart that illustrates the relationship between different hormones and use it to explain to your fellow students how each hormone influences the lactation course. (S)

10. Compare breastfeeding and bottle-feeding for each of the elements identified in TR 4-8 and 4-9. (S)
    a. In each case, how does failure to acknowledge these differences contribute to assumptions about feeding and health equivalence between infant feeding methods?
    b. What is the importance for the clinician of these differences?
    c. How might acceptance of breastfeeding as normal affect current clinical practices, beliefs, and attitudes, particularly as they relate to neonatal assessment and care giving?

11. Why are the differences between infant and adult oral anatomy important? (Refer to TR 4-10, 4-11). (I)

Chapter 5

The Biologic Specificity of Breastmilk

Breastmilk, like all other milks, is species-specific—a perfect "match" to the needs of the human infant. Although components of human milk remain relatively stable through lactation, subtle changes correspond to the child's maturation. Breastfeeding is health promotion and disease prevention in its purest form. Immunologic protection from acute infections, allergies, and chronic diseases is now recognized. Informed consent for pregnant women considering how they will feed their baby must include the health benefits of breastfeeding and the risks of not breastfeeding.

KEY CONCEPTS

Antiallergenic properties - Breastfeeding protects infants from allergies. Where milk is regularly consumed, bovine milk is the most common allergen. Milk processing has reduced but not eliminated allergies from bovine proteins.

Antibacterial and antiviral protection - Human milk contains leukocytes, lactoferrin, factor, lactoperoxidase, and complement that create an inhospitable environment for harmful bacteria and viruses.

Anti-inflammatory components- Anti-inflammatory components in breastmilk aid in the infant's defense against infectious disease.

Composition of human milk - Fat content provides about one-half of the calories in human milk; lactose is the predominate carbohydrate. Human milk protein is about one-half that of bovine milk and includes many immunological properties and all ten essential amino acids. Breastmilk supplies all vitamin and mineral requirements. Children at risk for rickets should be given Vitamim D supplements.

Epidermal growth factor - EGF, a major growth-promoting agent in breastmilk, stimulates growth of mucosal cells and epithelium, and is also present in other body fluids.

Hormones - Prostaglandins, cortisol, and thyrotropin-releasing hormone are ancillary components that help protect the infant against infections and disease. The function of hormones in human milk is still under investigation.

Immunoglobulins - There are five types of immunoglobulins: IgG, IgA, IgM, IgE, and IgD. Both IgA and IgE are critical in providing immune protection.

Infant growth - Breastfed and artificially-fed infants grow at about the same rate until the fourth month. After this point non-breastfed babies tend to grow faster. At one year of age, there are few differences in weight based upon feeding method. Breastfed infants have lower energy requirements and consume fewer kilocalories than non-breastfed babies.

Milk volume - Milk volume varies widely from woman to women and is limited only by intake needs of the infant. Volume may range from 200 to 3500 mL/day. The average breastmilk volume per day at one month postpartum is about 600 to 900 mL if the mother is exclusively breastfeeding.

READINGS FOR FURTHER REFERENCE

Lawrence, R. *Breastfeeding: A Guide for the Medical Profession.* St. Louis: C.V. Mosby, 4th edition, 1994. See esp. Chapters 4 and 5.

Neville, MC, Neifert, MR, Eds.*Lactation: Physiology, Nutrition, and Breast-Feeding.* New York; Plenum Press, 1983. See esp. Chapters 7 and 8.

Walker, M. A fresh look at the risks of artificial infant feeding. *J Hum Lact* 9: 97-107, 1993.

LEARNING ACTIVITIES

1. Talk to a pathologist or an epidemiologist (or bring one to class). Ask her/him to discuss the most common causes of death in the neonatal or postneonatal period. Which of these causes of death might be related to how an infant is fed? (I)

2. (Refer to TR 5-3). How is knowledge of breastmilk volume important for: (I)
   a. mothers
   b. health care workers
   In what way, might such knowledge be misused? an aid in assessing appropriate growth?

3. What maturational changes occur in human milk over time and what is their significance? (I)

4. Review the different nutritional elements in human milk. Compare them to that which is found in artificial baby milks. (I,S)

5. Explain how the anti-inflammatory elements in human milk work to support optimal infant health. (I,S)

6. Review how the energy levels of human milk change over time and from the beginning to the end of a feeding. Explain why human milk changes in volume and caloric level are important to the infant and young child's growth and development (refer to TR 5-2). (I,S)

7. Review the anti-infective properties of human milk and explain how you would inform a mother about these properties and why they are important to her own health and to her baby's health (refer to TR 5-3). (S)

8. Invite a group of four lactation consultants to class and explain what they share with mothers about the following topics: (I)
   a. milk volume and caloric capacity
   b. nutritional elements in human milk
   c. anti-infective properties
   d. immune system
   e. bioactive elements of human milk
   f. anti-allergenic properties of human milk

9. Compare and contrast the likelihood of infant illness by feeding groups. Write a paper based on the research of a minimum of 10 recent articles from the professional literature that assesses infant morbidity from a particular illness. (S)

CHAPTER 6

Drugs and Breastfeeding

Numerous factors influence whether a drug will have no, a beneficial, or adverse effect on the person taking it. Some factors are maternal in origin; others relate to the infant; and, still others relate to the bioactivity of the drug itself. This chapter examines the relationship between pharmaceuticals and environmental contaminants and their effect on lactating women, the milk they produce, and the infant receiving that milk.

KEY CONCEPTS

Addiction - The physiologic or psychologic dependence on some agent or agents which results in a tendency to increase its use to potentially short-term and/or long-term life-threatening levels.

Drug Diffusion - The movement of an agent from a higher to a lower concentration. One can illustrate this concept by pouring a small amount of dye into a large beaker of water and observing the change from deep (concentrated) color to a much paler hue as the dye mixes and thus is of a lower concentration in the beaker of water.

Environmental Contaminants - Usually refers to the existence, and concentration, of elements that are manufactured and which in sufficient concentrations represent risk of toxicity to other living forms, including plant and animal life. Common elements within this class include organochlorines, biphenyls, and radioactive elements.

Feeding Frequency - How often in a given time period an infant or adult ingests food.

"Guilty unless proven innocent" - A concept whereby human milk is assumed to be contaminated by one or more elements the mother has ingested in the absence of proof that such contamination has—indeed—occurred.

Half-life - The time period required for the level of original radioactivity of a given isotope to be reduced by half as a result of radioactive decay.

Infant age/maturity - A factor in the relative risk or potential for harm when a breastfeeding infant is exposed to a maternally-ingested drug.

Lipid soluble - A property by which elements are bound to fat molecules and thus passed from mother to infant via the lipid molecules in the mother's milk.

Metabolism of a Drug - The factors specific to a given drug which govern its bioactivity.

Milk/Plasma Ratio - The relative concentration of protein-free fractions of a drug in milk and in plasma. Concentrations may be high or low in milk or plasma, the same in both fluids, or higher in milk than in plasma.

Molecular Weight - The weight of a molecule of a given substance compared with that of the weight of an atom of carbon-12. The molecular weight of a drug is one factor contributing to the drug's likelihood of transmission from the mother into her milk. The higher the molecular weight (above 200), the lower the likelihood of such transfer.

Route of Administration - The means by which a drug is given (via injection, orally, or topically).

READINGS FOR FURTHER REFERENCE

DeLallo D, et al: Radioactivity in breast milk in Central Italy in the aftermath of Chernobyl. *Acta Paediatr Scand* 76:530-31, 1987

Gori G, et al: Radioactivity in breast milk and placentas during the year after Chernobyl. *Am J Obstet Gynecol* 159:1232-34, 1988

Lindemann R, Christensen GC: Radioactivity in breastmilk after the Chernobyl accident (letter). *Acta Paediatr Scand* 76:981-86, 1987

LEARNING ACTIVITIES

1. Describe addiction. Provide examples that illustrate the effect of a particular addicting drug on the lactating mother, on her breastfeeding infant. (I, S)

2. Explain how the principle of drug diffusion is affected by milk production and the transfer of milk from the mother's breast to the infant. (I)

3. Distinguish between the health-promoting/sustaining use of radioactive compounds and their concentration such that these same compounds are classified an environmental contaminant. If using the Chernobyl articles as an example, explain the food chain differences in level of risk of exposure. (I, S)

4. How is feeding frequency related to drug ingestion and its relative risk to the breastfeeding infant? In what way(s) might medication use be altered to reduce the infant's risk of exposure? (S)

5. How might "guilty unless proven innocent" be used as an argument against drug use? How might the concept be refuted when the question "drug or breastmilk" is raised? (S)

6. Examine the variation of half-lives of three or more radioactive substances sometimes prescribed for breastfeeding women. In each case, what does information regarding the half-life of a particular radioactive drug mean as it relates to breastfeeding? (I)

7. Explain how the solubility of a drug can influence its likelihood of a) transfer, and b) concentration in human milk, and c) the breastfeeding infant. (I, S)

8. Review the six drug factors noted in TR 6- 1. Explain how each can affect the pregnant woman, her fetus, the lactating mother, her milk, and the breastfeeding infant. (I)

9. Explain the milk/plasma ratio. Provide two examples of the M/P ratio in each of the following cases: (S)
   a. M/P ratio is very low
   b. M/P ratio is 1.0
   c. M/P ratio is very high
   In each case, what implications relative to breastfeeding are present and how might one change the M/P ratio to reduce the potential concentration of the drug in human milk?

10. Identify the molecular weights of three drugs whose weight is: a) <200; b) >200. In each case, what is the likelihood of finding the drug in...? (I)
    a. human milk
    b. maternal plasma
    c. infant plasma
    What do those findings tell us about the relative "safety" of using the drug during lactation?

11. Explain how the route of administration of a drug will influence its likelihood of transmission from the lactating mother to her breastfeeding baby. (I,S)

Chapter 7

Viruses in human milk

Antibodies in breastmilk augment the infants' passive immunity against viral infections and are an important method of child immunization. Breastfeeding may continue when either the mother or infant have a viral infection excepting a maternal HIV positive status and where the mother has a herpes simplex lesion on her breast.

KEY CONCEPTS

Chickenpox - An acute communicable disease that may be seen in the breastfeeding mother or her infant. Breastfeeding may continue in nearly all cases.

Cytomegalovirus - Breastfeeding is an important means of conveying passive immunity to cytomegalovirus to the infant. This immunity protects the child later in life from infection, and is particularly important during pregnancy.

Hepatitis B - Infants born to an HBV-positive mother are already exposed during delivery and may breastfeed. The neonate should receive Hepatitis B Immune Globulin soon after birth and in two subsequent injections.

Herpes simplex - Painful muco-cutaneous blister-like vesicles caused by the herpes virus that can erupt anywhere on the body including the breast or genital area. Direct contact with lesions should be avoided. When the mother has a lesion on her breast, she should interrupt breastfeeding and express her milk.

Human immumodeficiency virus (HIV) - At the time of this writing it is standard advice in Western medicine that no HIV-infected woman should breastfeed.

Passive immunity - Immunity conferred on an infant by antibodies manufactured by the mother and passed to the infant transplacentally or in breastmilk. Passive immunity is temporary as opposed to active immunity, which is lifelong.

Rubella - Transmission of maternal antibodies against rubella is beneficial to the infant by servig as a natural vaccine.

Seroconversion - When antibodies to an infecting agent such as cytomegalovirus or human immunodeficiency virus are present in the serum, the person is said to have seroconverted.

TORCH - Acronym for toxoplasmosis, rubella, cytomegalovirus, and herpes.

Viral transmission - Several viruses such as cytomegalovirus, rubella and HIV are thought to pass through human milk. This transmission is considered to have protective effects except in the case of HIV.

READING FOR FUTHER REFERENCE

Fekety, S. Managing the HIV-positive patient and her newborn in a CNM service. *J Nurse Midwif* 34: 253-58, 1989.

Pass, RF. Viral contamination of milk. *In* Goldman, AS, Atkinson, SA, Hanson A, eds.: *Human Lactation 3: The Effects of Milk on Recipient Infant.* New York: Plenum Press, 1986, pp. 279-87.

LEARNING ACTIVITIES

1. Write a paper that summarizes recent (published in the last three years) research on HIV and breastfeeding. Present this information to the class and distribute the reference list. Lead a discussion on the pro's and con's of breastfeeding when the mother is HIV+ based on the summarized findings of the studies. Explain under what circumstances your recommendations might be altered. (S)

2. Contact one or more health care professionals who work with mothers and infants who are at risk for developing AIDS. Interview them in depth to gather qualitative information about their experiences working with these families. Before the interview develop a list of open-ended questions to ask them. Write a paper on the findings. (S)

3. Explain passive immunity. Contrast it with active immunity. For what illnesses are immunizations or oral preparations available and when are they likely to be administered to infants/young children? How would such immunization (in each case) affect the breastfeeding infant? (I, S)

4. Review how viruses work and their effect on health. (I)

5. Review which viruses (I,S)
   a. are transmitted through human milk
   b. are likely to be less serious in the breastfeeding baby, and why
   c. require interruption or cessation of breastfeeding
   d. do not require interruption of breastfeeding.

6. Discuss each of the viruses listed in TR 7-1. In each case, note: (I)
   a. what data support the recommendation pertaining to breastfeeding
   b. the clinical significance of the recommendations pertaining to breastfeeding.

CHAPTER 8

Breastfeeding Education

This chapter focuses on the principles of adult education and how they are applied to breastfeeding education, both for parents and for professionals. How change is facilitated in the course of providing continuing education is discussed, as are a variety of ways in which to "capture" an audience so that new knowledge about lactation and/or breastfeeding may serve as the impetus for improved clinical practice.

KEY CONCEPTS

1. **Adult education** - Activities and approaches that facilitate learning in adults. Such approaches are most effective when they include opportunities to share related experiences and to be viewed as active participants in the learning environment.

2. **Breastfeeding education** - that teaching-learning opportunity that focuses attention on breastfeeding skills which are imparted within the context of information about the lactation course or process. Breastfeeding education may be provided in grade school, high school, as part of mother-to-mother support groups, in college classes, during prenatal and early postnatal contacts with young families, and throughout the breastfeeding course.

3. **Change process** - the process by which previous actions, routines, or other behaviors are altered as a result of an awareness of need, and following plans that incorporate new actions, routines or other behaviors.

4. **Continuing education** - a form of information sharing that is designed to assist persons specific to their occupation or profession. Such opportunities to learn new knowledge and new skills often are offered at the work site and often, during regular work hours. Other offerings, while of similar length, are offered off-site and may vary in length from a few hours to several days. Most professions now consider continuing education to be essential in enabling practitioners to remain current with new practice skills and understanding.

5. **Curriculum development** - the means by which all educational programs structure what will be taught and how it will be presented. Particularly as it relates to adult continuing education, needs assessment by the participating learner is considered a crucial first step in developing curricula.

6. **Infant feeding decision** - in societies where a baby will die in the absence of access to mother's milk, the decision to breastfeed is cleart. It is less clear in settings where alternatives do not kill the majority of its recipients. In such a setting, infant feeding decisions are often made on the basis of social, rather than infant survival, considerations. In such a setting, the more informed the person is about the benefits and risks of different feeding options, the more likely the mother is to breastfeed.

7. **Learner objectives** - those elements in an educational program that describe one or more rationale for including certain elements in the education program.

8. **Learning principles** - those elements that govern the student's interest in seeking new knowledge and/or skills. Such principles also govern the

techniques considered most appropriate for a given group of students and/or in a given setting.

9. **Parent education** - opportunities to teach skills or impart information specific to the parenting experience. These topics may include material oriented to maternal or paternal behavior or specific to infancy and childhood of the children of the parent learners.

10. **Practical information** - that knowledge or those skills that can be applied in everyday life.

11. **Small group dynamics** - the interaction of a group changes as the group adds or subtracts members. In addition, the skills and presentation of self of the members influences how well the group works as a team.

12. **Teaching strategies** - the techniques used to impart new information and/or new skills or skills based on previous understandings and skills. Such strategies will be most effective when the needs of the group are most closely met by the techniques the teacher uses to involve the students in the learning experience.

13. **Team approach** - both teaching and learning can occur within the context of group experiences. Team teaching uses more than one teacher, thereby taking advantage of the complementary skills and approaches of more than one leader. Team learning requires that the participants work together to achieve closure of the task at hand.

14. **Therapeutic communication** - includes a variety of techniques that may supercede verbal communication. These include non-language use of the voice, body motion/posture and/or gestures, touch, and the like. Therapeutic communication may also include verbal techniques such as reflecting, restating, and paraphrasing another's statements in order to clarify and validate her or his views. Techniques of therapeutic communication are designed to assist or enhance communication.

READINGS FOR FURTHER REFERENCE

Bocar DL, Moore K: *Acquiring the Parental Role : A Theoretical Perspective* (Unit 16). Lactation Consultant Series. Garden City Park, NY: Avery Publishing Group, 1987.

Boyd MA: Communication with patients, families, healthcare providers, and diverse cultures. In Strader MK, Decker, PJ: *Role Transition to Patient Care Management*. Englewood Cliffs, NJ: Appletone and Lange, 1995.

Leddy S, Pepper, JM: The process of teaching-learning (Chapter 15). *Conceptual Bases of Professional Nursing* . Philadelphia: JB Lippincott, 1993.

Valaitis R, O'Brien MF: A local community's approach to breastfeeding promotion. *J Hum Lact* 10:113-18, 1994.

LEARNING ACTIVITIES

1. Contrast adult education with the kind of teaching often employed when working with children. (I)

2. Ask your students to observe an adult education class in which they are not student/ teacher participants. They should then characterize the kind of education that occurred and how it differs from that offered to children or adolescents. (S)

3. Ask your students to select two of the following settings to observe and then describe breastfeeding education. The emphasis of their description should include identification of similarities and differences between the two settings: (S)
   a. Prenatal breastfeeding class (in community)
   b. Postnatal breastfeeding class (in hospital)
   c. Class discussing breastfeeding in junior high school
   d. Class discussing breastfeeding in high school
   e. Class discussing breastfeeding in college (any class)
   f. Mother-to-mother support group (in community)

4. Identify several elements that would be considered appropriate breastfeeding education. (I)

5. Distinguish between the anticipatory, formal, informal, and personal stages of role acquisition to parenthood. (See Bocar and Moore.) Note how these stages will influence parenting education. (I)

6. Distinguish between the change process as put forth by Lewin, Rogers, Havelock and Lippitt (see TR8-1, 8-2, 8-3). (I)

7. Ask the students to critique the change process as described by Valaitis and O'Brien. Ask them to compare the process of forming, storming, norming, performing, and adjourning to other stages of change already presented. (S)

8. Form your students into groups and develop a "model" one-hour continuing education program with some aspect of breastfeeding as the topic. The program will then be presented to another group of students and critiqued for its effectiveness in presenting new information. (S)

9. Have each student develop a one-hour continuing education program for a group of professionals of her/his choosing. The participants' critiques are to be used as the basis for the students' self-assessment of the effectiveness of the program in presenting new information. (S)

10. Present the same information to illustrate each of the following aspects of curriculum content: (I)
    a. chronological
    b. utilization
    c. simple to complex
    d. general to specific
    e. known to unknown

11. Ask your students to develop an outline for a curriculum using two of the following aspects of curriculum content: (S)
    a. chronological
    b. utilization
    c. simple to complex
    d. general to specific
    e. known to unknown

12. Discuss how infant feeding decisions can be influenced by educational offerings (see TR 8-4). (I)

13. Ask the students to develop an outline of a continuing education offering. Their outline should include a title, brief description of the program, and 3-5 objectives. (S)

14. Discuss the five learning principles shown on TR 8-4. (I)

15. Have your students outline a parent education class on any topic of their choosing. The following elements need to be included in their outline? (S)
    a. emotional responses to the topic
    b. previous personal experiences relating to the topic
    c. three practical aspects of care related to the topic

16. Distinguish between a theoretical discussion and one that focuses on practical information on one or more of the following topics: (I)
    a. discipline
    b. day care
    c. breastfeeding
    d. introducing solid foods
    e. weaning
    f. toilet training
    g. teaching breastfeeding

17. Break the students into small groups with the following dimensions: (S)
    a. 2-person group
    b. 3-person group
    c. 4-person group
    d. 5-person group
    Ask each group to discuss the same topic. Have one other student (not a member of the group) observe and report on the dynamics of each group's structure (who talked, who didn't, who asked questions, who answered, and the like). Compare the observations through discussion by the entire class. (S)

18. Identify at least four different teaching strategies and how each might contribute to an effective learning experience. (I)

19. Have the students break into teams of two or three persons and collectively develop a presentation about some aspect of breastfeeding. As part of their paper describing their experience, they will discuss the pros and cons of the team approach to the project. (S)

20. Describe therapeutic communicaton and how it differs from other kinds of information-sharing. (I)

21. Invite a practitioner of therapeutic touch to visit the class and demonstrate techniques and why they have been found effective. (I)

22. In what way(s) might each of the communication techniques listed in TR 8-5 contribute to: (I,S)
    a. prenatal decision-making pertaining to infant feeding
    b. early postnatal decision-making pertaining to infant feeding
    c. late postnatal decision-making pertaining to infant feeding
    d. anticipatory decision-making for a future baby/child.

CHAPTER 9

The Breastfeeding Process

This chapter reviews the early breastfeeding period and common concerns pertaining to the hospitalization period and early weeks of lactation. Feeding techniques and clinical concerns pertaining to preparation for early discharge are given special attention.

KEY CONCEPTS

1. **Breast Fullness** - An experience of early lactation in which the mother experiences generalized swelling of the breast tissue, but not sufficiently to prevent milk transfer or compressibility of the breast tissue by the neonate.

2. **Breast Refusal** - Reaction of the baby to the mother's offer of the breast. In most cases, this behavior occurs after the baby is six months old; when it occurs earlier, the behavior may reflect a preference for rubber teat/nipple feedings when the baby is learning how to breastfeed or a learned aversive reaction to being forced to take the breast.

3. **Discharge planning** - The means by which the health care worker assists the mother as she leaves the birth-site confident in her ability to continue to mother her newborn. Ideally, discharge planning meets two goals: prevention of commonly-occurring problems and provision of emotional support.

4. **Engorgement** - An experience of early lactation such that the infant may not be able to suckle and/or milk transfer may be inhibited. In many cases, women are informed that engorgement is a sign of early lactation. If, however, they are not informed how to reduce the negative effects of engorgement, they may experience unnecessary difficulty that can contribute to other related problems, including infant frustration, maternal nipple and breast pain and trauma, and the like.

5. **Feeding Plan** - a plan for optimal care that identifies the parents' wishes in advance of the baby's birth to focus discussion with the health providers regarding how the mother wishes her baby's right to her own milk to be preserved, protected, and supported.

6. **Hypoglycemia** - a deficiency, usually temporary, of blood glucose. In the infant's first 24 hours, hypoglycemia is defined as a blood glucose level less than 30 mg/dL. In later days, it is defined as less than 40 mg/dL. In many cases where a mother has had an intravenous glucose drip during a portion, or all, of her labor, the baby's glucose levels will drop more steeply when the maternal drip is no longer a source of additional glucose in the baby.

7. **Insufficient milk supply** - A world-wide perception harbored by many women that they are not producing, or are unable to produce, enough milk to meet their baby's needs. Far fewer women are proven to be physiologically unable to produce sufficient milk than believe it to be the case.

8. **Leaking** - an experience usually limited to the first month of the early breastfeeding course and times when overfullness occurs in which milk may drip or spurt from the contralateral breast while the infant is suckling the other breast, or from both breasts when the infant is not breastfeeding. In most cases, such leaking does not continue throughout the

breastfeeding period and it is easily controlled by a brief period (5-10 seconds) of gentle pressure.

9. **Massage** - A technique, when applied to the breast, that is used to resolve a variety of temporary conditions, including engorgement, plugged ducts, mastitis, and/or to increase milk transfer. Its use varies in different culture.

10. **Multiple infants** - a term used to refer to the birth and nurturing of more than one infant at the same time; e.g., twins, triplets, quadruplets, and quintuplets.

11. **Sore nipples** - One of the most common transient problems reported by breastfeeding mothers. Although not yet rigorously evaluated, how the baby feeds appears to be an important antecedent to nipple soreness; other factors previously considered to contribute to nipple soreness; e.g., skin complexion, duration of suckling episodes, have not held up to rigorous research-based scrutiny.

12. **Stooling** - Stooling patterns of breastfed babies vary from that observed in artificially-fed infants. In most cases, these differences are not cause for concern; however, caregivers should be aware of these differences so as not to alarm the mother unnecessarily and to appropriately identify when the pattern of stooling indicates the need for careful additional evaluation of the feeding course.

13. **Suckling pattern** - A well-organized sequence of behaviors that stimulates milk production and ejection in the mother when the baby breastfeeds. The suckling pattern includes a rhythmic suck-swallow-breathe response that varies from rapid to slow to rapid during the course of the suckling episode.

READINGS FOR FURTHER REFERENCE

Baranowski, T, Bee, DE, Rassin, DK, et al: Social support, social influence, ethnicity and the breast-feeding decision. *Soc Sci Med* 17:1599-1611, 1983.

Buckner, E, Matsubara, M: Support network utilization by breastfeeding mothers. *J Hum Lact* 9:231-35, 1993.

Hill, PD, Humenick, SS: The occurrence of breast engorgement. *J Hum Lact* 10:79-86, 1994.

Hill, PD, Humenick, SS, Anderson, MA: Breast engorgement: patterns and selected outcomes. *J Hum Lact* 10:87-93, 1994.

Moon, JL, Humenick, SS: Breast engorgement: contributing variables and variables amenable to nursing intervention. *JOGNN* 18:309-15, 1989.

Mulford C: The mother-baby assessment (MBA): an "Apgar score" for breastfeeding. *J Hum Lact* 8:79-82, 1992.

Saunders, SE, Carroll, J: Post-partum breast feeding support: impact on duration. *J Am Diet Assoc* 88:213-15, 1988.

Serafino-Cross, P, Donovan, PR: Effectiveness of professional breastfeeding home support. *Soc Nutr Educ* 24:117-22, 1992.

LEARNING ACTIVITIES

1. Review the differences between engorgement and breast fullness (see TR 9-1.) (I)

2. Ask the students to read the work of Humenick and Hill (both articles in additional references). Ask them to explain how they would define breast fullness based on these new findings. Ask them to justify their definition. (S)

3. Distinguish the different factors that are likely to result in infant breast refusal shortly after birth, and after six months of age. (I)

4. On the blackboard, label two columns: "preventing common problems" and "providing emotional support." Ask the students to identify elements relevant to each column. (I)

5. Review the pros and cons of early discharge from the birth site. (I)
   a. What is "early discharge?" What is "late discharge?" How have these terms changed since the 1940s?
   b. How might "early discharge" vary in its definition in different countries? Give at least three examples.
   c. Explain how telephone follow-up and home visits may mitigate against some of the negative aspects of early discharge.

6. Divide the students into three groups: one group will identify what a new mother should know—prior to hospital discharge—about positioning; another group will focus on basic feeding techniques; and the third group will focus on signs that intervention is needed. (S)
   a. Following their in-class discussion, each student in each group will interview 5 mothers, asking them what they were taught prior to hospital discharge about the subject on which their group focused.
   b. At the conclusion of these interviews, the students will compare what they identified as appropriate with the information the mothers reported having received.

7. Use at least two different visual aids to identify the size of a newborn's stomach. Ask the students to ask mothers how large they think their baby's stomach is and how much milk the baby should be able to take each feeding. Ask the students to compare the assumptions of breastfeeding and artificially-feeding mothers. How might these differences contribute to misunderstandings regarding neonatal needs? (I/S)

8. Contrast differences between the recommendations: "offer both breasts at each feeding" and "finish the first breast first." How might mothers have difficulty with each admonition? How might the health worker advise the mother in order to reduce confusion or a sense that there is only "one right way" to breastfeed? (I)

9. Review the seven signs that intervention is needed, identify at least one clinical problem indicative of each sign and how intervention might resolve the problem while preserving the breastfeeding course. (I)

10. Ask the students to review the positive and negative elements related to each of three positioning options as seen in Table 9-6. Using mother interviews, ask the students to select the order with which they would teach positioning that enhances positive aspects and minimizes their negative effects. Of each mother, the students should ask... (S)
    a. what position(s) were the mothers taught in hospital? by whom?
    b. If the mothers were taught more than one position, which were they taught first?
    c. If they were not taught about positioning, what position did they choose to use? Did they develop sore nipples? If so, how long did they last? How was this problem (if experienced) resolved?
    d. What did the mothers know about positioning before the baby's birth?
    e. How did the mother's comfort with infant positioning options change after the baby's birth?
    f. What position does the mother prefer to use now? Why? If this is a position different from the first one she used, what factor(s) contributed to the change of positions that she now uses?
    g. If the mothers received contradictory advice regarding positioning, who said/recommended what? Why? What was the outcome?

11. Discuss the importance of post-discharge support. (I)
    a. Compare the availability of such care in different cultures (see articles by Baranowski, Buckner, Saunders, and Serafino-Cross).
    b. Discuss the problems that can arise when no such assistance is available.
    c. How is post-discharge support currently provided in the US? How might such support be made more widely available?

12. Ask the students to review Humenick and Hill's characterization of breast engorgement patterns. In interviews with five women, ask the students to characterize the *kind* of engorgement each woman described. The mothers should be asked for enough detail to justify the characterization that the student will report in each case. Ask the students to provide a conclusion regarding the likelihood of engorgement as a result of their interviews and the information they obtained. If a woman states that she never experienced engorgement, ask the student to explain why the mother felt she had no engorgement, and how this experience might influence what the mother might tell other mothers. (S)

13. Review the Moon and Humenick reference. Explain why some variables have an inverse relationship and why others have a positive relationship to the likelihood of breast engorgement in the postpartal period. Explain how you might improve on this study with a later investigation, and why. (I)

14. Review the feeding plan provided in Chapter 9. For at least two local birth sites, identify how much of this feeding plan could be implemented without changing current institutional routines and practices. (I)

15. Ask the students to observe how infants are fed in one or more local birth settings. Ask them to inquire about each of the elements in the feeding plan offered in Chapter 9. (S)
    a. How many elements are currently available to breastfeeding mothers and their babies?
    b. Which elements are not yet available?
    c. For those elements identified in (b) above, what reaction to each element have the students observed when interviewing at least five different staff members working at that birth site (encourage the students to interview at least one person from each of the following groups: physician, midwife, nurse) regarding the appropriateness of providing such an option?
    d. The students should review what they have learned and prioritize each of the nine elements in the birth plan regarding what is currently available and regularly practiced, and what is not yet practiced but could be incorporated (easiest/least disliked to most difficult to implement). Justification for the ordering of elements should be required.

16. Ask several local hospital representatives to discuss the implications of the feeding plan provided in Chapter 9 from the perspective of their role. Persons invited to sit on such a panel might include: (I)
    a. an obstetrician
    b. a pediatrician
    c. a family practice physician
    d. a nurse who cares for mothers and their babies in the hospital
    e. a midwife
    f. a community-based lactation consultant whose clients use the hospital in question

17. Ask the students to identify what level of blood glucose is used as a marker for hypoglycemia in neonates in at least two local hospitals. Then ask the students to determine: (S)
    a. how blood glucose levels are measured
    b. when blood glucose levels are measured
    c. how often blood glucose levels are measured
    d. how heel stick measures are confirmed?
    e. routine treatment for breastfeeding babies who are determined to be hypoglycemic

18. Review the eight elements noted for helping a mother with early breastfeedings. Ask the students to pair off and use a doll to simulate the early breastfeeding experience. Taking turns, each student "role plays" mother while the other "role plays" helping caregiver. Each then shares with the other how she felt as she sought to bring her baby to breast. (S)

19. Identify situations when neonatal blood glucose levels are likely to be considered a cause for concern. (I)

20. Review the reasons given by Walker (1989) [Transparency 2] related to infant behavior or maternal experiences that lead many women to conclude that they do not have sufficient milk. In each case, explain how the mother might conclude that she does not have sufficient milk and how such a conclusion may be based on one or more false assumptions. (I)

21. Examine each cluster of elements pertaining to insufficient milk supply shown in TR 9-2, 9-3). Ask the students to explain how each element within each cluster may relate, respectively, to a direct or indirect influence on milk production. (I/S)

22. Review when and why women are likely to experience leaking. (I)

23. Review how breast massage is used in different cultures. Compare its use in the U.S. with other settings. (I)

24. Review some of the common difficulties mothers of multiples experience in hospital and how they can be resolved. (I)

25. Review the four assessment questions related to nipple soreness that are discussed in Chapter 9 (see TR 9-4). Provide live examples of each with breastfeeding mother and babies or videos of same. (I)

26. Review factors found *not* to be associated with nipple soreness. (I)

27. Demonstrate how the students can determine if the baby is properly or improperly positioned on the breast and how this might be related to sore nipples. [For example, see Delivery Self Attachment film listed in AV Resources.] (S)

28. Review the list of items on pp.232-33 of Chapter 9. How many of these items are used (or distributed) in at least two different hospitals in the local community? How many are available, and at what price, in drug stores, pharmacies, and other outlets available to the general public? What recommendations would the class recommend to breastfeeding mothers with whom they might come in contact? (I)

29. Encourage the students to develop a research proposal based on the clinical care plan for sore nipples, whose aim is to test the hypothesis that positioning the baby appropriately on the breast will reduce or prevent the occurrence of sore nipples. (S)

30. Review the information about stool patterns over time in Table 9-5. Refer to this information when comparing what might be expected of a baby who is being fed artificial baby milk. Explain how the pattern of the artificially-fed baby might generate concern in an uninformed breastfeeding mother. (I)

31. Using the Matthews IBFAT (see Chapter 21), describe infant suckling behavior. Explain how this tool might be used to assess how well or poorly the baby is contributing to an ample milk supply. (I)

32. Ask the students to compare use of the IBFAT with the MBA as developed by Mulford. Which of these tools would they recommend; under what circumstances? (S)

CHAPTER 10

Breastfeeding and the Pre-Term Infant

This chapter examines the effect of premature birth on the mother's lactation course and on her infant's ability to breastfeed and subsequent feeding patterns that are likely to occur as a result of early birth.

KEY CONCEPTS

1. **Bacteriologic surveillance** - protocols designed to reduce the number of potentially pathogenic organisms found in expressed human milk. This issue pertains to preterm and other compromised neonates who are unlikely to obtain milk directly from the breast.

2. **Breastfeeding management** - for preterm infants, management of breastfeeding may involve gavage or other means of feeding, feeding directly from the breast, and the necessary steps in between. In-hospital as well as post-discharge feeding patterns need to be individualized to meet the needs of each mother-infant pair.

3. **Expressed mother's milk** - any milk the mother obtains from her breasts by whatever technique in order to give milk to her baby who may be unable to obtain it directly from her breasts.

4. **Expression schedule** - the frequency and timing of episodes of daily milk expression that a mother uses in order to maintain her milk supply during the period when her baby is unable to suckle directly.

5. **Feedings from different containers** - when a baby cannot feed from the breast, other techniques may be needed to feed the infant. These techniques can include bottle, cups, or a variety of tube feeding methods. In all cases, the care provider must remain sensitive to the differences between such techniques and direct breastfeeding.

6. **Gavage feeding** - one technique for providing milk to the preterm infant. Gavage feeding may be by continuous infusion or intermittent infusion. With continuous infusion, feedings are subject to other problems such as greater loss of the lipid portion and higher bacterial contamination of the milk, even though continuous drip is less subject to the creation of adverse short-term problems such as apnea, bradycardia, and hypoxemia.

7. **Human milk fortifiers** - commercial products designed to be added to human milk to increase caloric density of the milk in order to enhance growth. Other macronutrients such as calcium and phosphorus can also be increased with the use of such fortifiers with preterm mother's milk.

8. **Test-weighings** - measuring milk transfer by pre- and post-feed infant weights. Only accurate electronic scales should be used and coupled with assistance and reassurance of the mother regarding the meaning of such weighings.

READINGS FOR FURTHER REFERENCE

Hill, PD, Hanson, KS, Mefford, AL: Mothers of low birthweight infants: breastfeeding patterns and problems. *J Hum Lact* 10:169-74, 1994.

Lang, S, Lawrence, CJ, Lé Orme, R: Cup feeding: an alternative method of infant feeding. *Arch Dis Child* 71:365-69, 1994.

Meier, P, Engstrom, JL, Mangurten, HH, et al: Breastfeeding support services in the neonatal intensive-care unit. *JOGNN* 22:338-47, 1993.

Walker, M, Driscoll, JW: *Breastfeeding Your Premature or Special Care Baby: A Practical Guide for Nursing the Tiny Baby*, 1989 (2nd ed.) 16 pages - illustrated - $5.50 + shipping. Orders: Lactation Associates, Weston, MA 02193-1756; 617-893-3553.

LEARNING ACTIVITIES

1. Review the rationale for bacteriologic surveillance of human milk for high-risk infants. (I)

2. Ask your students to inquire of at least three Level 3 hospitals what kind of bacteriologic surveillance techniques they employ to assure that expressed human milk is minimally contaminated. (S)

3. Refer to TR 10-1. Describe different techniques of breastfeeding management for preterm infants. Distinguish between in-hospital and post-discharge management. (I)

4. Discuss the step-by-step process for breastfeeding the premature infant as illustrated in TR 10-2. In what way(s) is it: (I)
   a. similar to breastfeeding a healthy term infant?
   b. different from breastfeeding a healthy term infant?

5. Ask your students to compare and contrast appropriate breastfeeding management for preterm infants with those for term infants. (S)

6. Review techniques for obtaining expressed mother's milk for use by preterm infants and discuss the risks and benefits of each technique. (I)

7. Ask mothers of preterm infants to share with the class their expression techniques and schedule. Be sure to ask them to note when and for how long they were able to obtain sufficient milk to meet their babies' needs. (I)

8. Ask your students to review the risks and benefits, as well as the frequency of use of feeding from different containers. This review can be an oral or written presentation. (S)

9. Describe gavage feeding. Have a neonatal nurse explain the problems with such feedings, which babies most benefit from it, and how to determine when such feedings are no longer necessary. (I)

10. Have a neonatologist describe the differences between currently available human milk fortifiers. Ask this expert to compare these fortifiers with the process of spinning down human milk and feeding hindmilk. (I)

CHAPTER 11

Breast Pumps and Other Technologies

This chapter reviews the creation and proliferation of devices designed to assist breastfeeding mothers. Ways to evaluate their appropriate use and their effects on the breastfeeding course also are discussed.

KEY CONCEPTS

1. **Breast Pump** - a device designed to obtain milk from a mother's breast in the absence of direct breastfeeding by the infant or hand expression by the mother. A wide variety of such devices is on the market, ranging from hand-operated to fully automatic electric items.

2. **Breast Shell** - a device worn at times other than during a breastfeeding episode; designed to evert an inverted nipple or to elongate a flat nipple. In some cases, breast shells are used to protect sore nipples from chafing by clothing.

3. **Feeding tube device** - a mechanism designed to provide nutriment to the infant while the baby is at the mother's breast. Several situations may be appropriate to the use of this device, including induced lactation, relactation, following breast surgery, when the mother has primary breast insufficiency, when attempting to reward a baby who has not yet associated breastfeeding with pleasure or food, and when a mother must temporarily provide additional nutriment to the infant. Most devices require careful instruction and observation of the mother and baby when the device is first used.

4. **Finger Feeding** - a technique whereby the baby is fed with a feeding tube or other device while sucking the finger of the caregiver or mother. Such a technique is considered by many to be less disruptive of the breastfeeding suckling pattern than bottle-feeding; others, however, express concerns about such a technique since it is not practiced in conjunction with direct breastfeeding.

5. **Milk Ejection Reflex** - The means by which milk is moved down the ducts and ductules of the breast into the nipple and thence into the baby's mouth. When using a breast pump or hand expression, milk ejection may be less efficient, erratic or delayed, insofar as both physiology and psychology play a role in an efficient milk ejection reflex.

6. **Nipple Shield** - a device that covers the human nipple and which is used to shape a flat nipple and/or to protect the sore or traumatized nipple from further damage during suckling. In some cases, a baby who has developed a preference for suckling a rubber nipple can be brought back to the breast with the judicious use of a nipple shield. A nipple shield may also harbor risks to the baby and, therefore, should be used with caution and careful follow-up.

READINGS FOR FURTHER REFERENCE

Auerbach, KG, Walker, M: When the mother of a premature infant uses a breast pump: what every NICU nurse needs to know. *Neonat Netw* 13:23-29, 1994.

Meier, PP, Engstrom, JL, Crichton, CL, et al: A new scale for in-home test-weighing for mothers of preterm and high risk infants. *J Hum Lact* 10:163-68, 1994.

LEARNING ACTIVITIES

1. Review six elements (see TR 11-1) mothers consider important in selecting a breast pump. Then determine as a class which breast pumps to recommend under specific circumstances. (I)

2. Invite a panel of mothers who are using a breast pump share their experiences with the class. Give them the list of recommendations and techniques (see TR11-2, 11-3) for breast pump use and ask—in each case—if they were instructed in each such recommendation (if so, by whom), and if not, what they were instructed to do instead. A short paper based on the students' observation of this panel might be a class assignment. (S)

3. Invite two breastfeeding mothers to attend the class. Then ask them to use, in sequence, at least five different breast pumps. Following each, they should share the following information with the class: (I)
   a. its efficiency (in five minutes, how much milk was obtained)
   b. her comfort when using the pump
   c. whether the mother became fatigued using the pump, and if so, what portion of her body became fatigued
   d. whether the mother would recommend the pump to others for occasional use, regular use if a baby is hospitalized (due to illness or prematurity), or regular use if the mother is employed fulltime outside the home.

4. Ask the students to develop a protocol for evaluating each class of breast pumps that is available (squeeze-handle pumps, for example) varieties of the same class of pumps compared against one another. The risks as well as the benefits of each pump should be emphasized. (S)

5. Review the concerns of professionals regarding the use of breast pumps (see TR 11-4). How do these concerns relate to those expressed by mothers (see #1 above)? (I)

6. Review the variations in design of breast shells. Bring samples to class and discuss how each might relate to maternal breast shape, comfort, and rationale for use. (I)

7. Review the prenatal and postpartum recommendations for use of breast shells. Ask mothers who have used them which recommendations, if any, they were given and, if so, by whom? (I)

8. Ask an LC to demonstrate the use and instruction of a feeding tube device, making sure to identify both the costs and benefits of the device. (I)

9. Ask a panel of mothers, each of whom has used a feeding tube device for a *different* reason, to share their experiences with the class. In each case, the mothers should be asked: (I)
   a. *why* did they use the feeding tube device?
   b. *who recommended* its use?
   c. *who instructed* her in its use?
   d. *how easy/difficult* did the mother find using the device?
   e. *why* did the mother feel this way?
   f. *how long* did the mother use the device?
   g. *what* did it *cost*? was it worth it?
   h. if more than one kind of feeding tube device was used, why was this?
   i. *what* would the mother recommend to other mothers who might be in the same situation as she?

10. Consider the use of a feeding-tube device compared to bottle-feeding, cup-feeding, and breastfeeding. In each case, identify the costs and benefits of each alternative when... (I)
    a. mother and baby are both in the hospital
    b. mother is home and baby is in the hospital
    c. mother is in the hospital and baby is at home
    d. the baby is premature
    e. the mother has primary breast insufficiency
    f. the baby is adopted

11. Review the reasons given (see TR 11-5, 11-6) for using a feeding tube device. What other options are available for each such situation? (I)

12. Review the "Instructions for Finger-Feeding a Neonate" (p. 222). Discuss how finger-feeding might: (I)
    a. complement breastfeeding
    b. serve as an alternative to breastfeeding
    c. interfere with direct breastfeeding

13. Review how the milk ejection reflex functions, what triggers it, what might inhibit it, and how breastfeeding and breast pumping differ regarding the milk ejection reflex. (I)

14. Review how nipple shields have changed over time. (I)

15. Review the reasons nipple shields are used (see TR 11-7). Consider alternative techniques that might be used instead of a nipple shield. (I)

CHAPTER 12

Jaundice and the Breastfeeding Baby

This chapter reviews early- and late-onset jaundice, how each affect continued breastfeeding and the most appropriate management of the breastfeeding infant who exhibits signs of hyperbilirubinemia.

KEY CONCEPTS

1. **Conjugated bilirubin** - sometimes called direct bilirubin, it is water soluble, and is excreted in the urine. Generally, water-soluble direct bilirubin poses no risk to the infant. If levels of direct bilirubin in serum are high, this may indicate biliary obstruction.

2. **Early-onset jaundice** - an elevation in serum bilirubin that is most likely to occur after the first 24 hours through the first week or longer of neonatal life. This condition poses no harm to the infant and represents an early adjustment to extrauterine life in an oxygen-rich environment; it requires no intervention.

3. **Incipient Vulnerable Child Syndrome** - A pattern of behavior expressed by parents who perceive that their child is at greater than expected risk for illness or death. At least one group of investigators has identified such behavior in parents whose neonate was diagnosed as "jaundiced" in the post-birth period of hospitalization.

4. **Late-onset jaundice** - A condition in which serum bilirubin levels are elevated after the first week of life. In most cases, the condition occurs in healthy, thriving infants; it requires no intervention after organic and functional problems, for which high serum bilirubin is a marker, have been ruled out.

5. **Non-human milk feeds** - any liquid derived from a concoction of ingredients produced with a non-human mammal milk or vegetable protein base that does not include human milk. Commercially manufactured baby milks are examples of such feeds.

6. **Pathologic jaundice** - a condition characterizing three general categories of concerns: diseases which cause increased red blood cell hemolysis (such as Rh disease, ABO incompatibility, congenital spherocytosis, or other hemolytic processes); carrier protein or binding deficiencies (such as prematurity, sepsis, hypoxia, or as a result of the use of certain drugs); or diseases of the liver or metabolism (such as hepatitis, Crigler-Najjar syndrome, Rotor's syndrome, liver damage from cytomegalovirus, toxoplasmosis, rubella, syphilis, congenital biliary atresia, galactosemia, hypothyroidism). In many cases, such pathologic jaundice resulting from liver disease or deficiencies of metabolism manifest themselves *after* the first week of life. Conditions causing red cell hemolysis or deficiencies of carrier protein or binding may manifest themselves as early as the first week of life and should be identified before recommending intervention.

7. **Serum bilirubin** - levels of bilirubin measured in the bloodstream. In most cases, early rises in serum bilirubin represent a normal adjustment to extrauterine life and require no intervention designed to result in an earlier-than-necessary decline in such levels.

8. **"Starvation-induced" jaundice** - the name given

to situations in which calorically-dense foods are withheld and/or delayed, or offered infrequently, thereby resulting in a rise in serum bilirubin levels. When neonates are fed sterile water (0 calories/oz) or glucose water(≈5-6 calories/oz) *in lieu of* breastfeeding freely, starvation-induced early-onset jaundice is the result. In contrast, access to sufficient calories in a milk preparation will coat the intestinal mucosa, thereby reducing the likelihood of reabsorption of unconjugated bilirubin.

9. **Unconjugated bilirubin** - sometimes called indirect bilirubin, that portion which is lipid (fat)-soluble and which is transported from the spleen to the liver through such transporting proteins as albumin. Unconjugated bilirubin is excreted in stool and is found in high concentrations in meconium. When the neonate is denied sufficient access to milk feedings, the unconjugated bilirubin may be recirculated through the liver rather than excreted, thereby resulting in an increase in the concentration of serum bilirubin.

10. **Water supplementation** - a practice whereby the neonate is fed water or glucose water in addition to or as a replacement for milk feeds. Such supplementation increases neither frequency nor volume of voids, but does reduce the frequency and volume of milk feeds and has been implicated in the etiology and duration of "starvation-induced" jaundice.

READINGS FOR FURTHER REFERENCE

Provisional Committee on Quality Improvement and Subcommitteee on Hyperbilirubinemia: Practice parameter: management of hyperbilirubinemia in the healthy term newborn. *Pediatrics* 94:558-65, 1994.

LEARNING ACTIVITIES

1. Review how bilirubin is transported to and broken down in the liver into its conjugated and unconjugated forms. How is eachexcreted and what are the implications of these differences for new parents? (I)

2. Identify early onset jaundice (see TR 12-1). For each of the seven elements noted in the "Summary of Characteristics of Early-Onset Jaundice," note what each characteristic means for ... (I)
   a. health care providers
   b. new parents
   c. newborn healthy infants.

3. Ask your students to observe how early onset jaundice is managed in at least two different hospitals. Ask them to describe each management pattern, paying particular attention to: (S)
   a. differences in management by hospital site
   b. differences in management by infant feeding method
   c. effect on parents of each observed management pattern
   d. effect on breastfeeding of each observed management pattern
   e. frequency of bili light therapy of each observed management pattern
   f. average cost per family of bilirubin management at each hospital

4. Define incipient vulnerable child syndrome; review how it can develop and how it might be avoided. Include in your discussion the effects of such a syndrome on short-term and long-term parenting patterns. (I)

5. Distinguish between early-onset and late-onset jaundice. (I)

6. Identify late-onset jaundice (see TR 12-2). For each of the nine elements noted in the "Summary of Characteristics of Late-Onset Jaundice," note what each characteristic means for... (I)
   a. health care providers
   b. new parents
   c. healthy infants.

7. Define non-human milk feeds. Distinguish between constituents of each of the following non-human milk feeds: cow milk-based fluids (two different brands); soy-protein based fluids (two different brands), lactose-free fluids (two different brands). To obtain the most accurate information not used as advertising copy, seek

information from sources independent of the marketing departments of the non-human milk proprietary companies. Discuss what elements are missing from each of these non-human milk feeds and the implications of their absence for optimal infant health. (I)

8. Define pathologic jaundice; discuss when it is most likely to occur and under what conditions. Distinguish between pathologic jaundice and early- and late-onset jaundice, and how the latter are often consi-dered diagnoses of elimination. (I)

9. Ask your students to explain how serum bilirubin is affected by specific infant factors and hospital routines. (S)

10. Explain how "starvation-induced" jaundice is caused and how it might be avoided (refer to TR 12-3). Relate its likelihood to occurrence of specific hospital rotuines and particular feeding recommendations. Explain how both artificially-fed and breastfed infants might be protected against its likelihood and the effects of "starvation-induced" jaundice. (I)

11. Relate water supplementation to other hospital routines pertaining to the feeding of newborns. (I)

CHAPTER 13

Maternal Health

Women of childbearing age are usually healthy. When chronic or infectious health problems develop in this population, they rarely require weaning the baby from the breast, but they do require caring assistance from the health care provider. Drug therapy that is compatible with breastfeeding is possible in almost all cases. Infection, alterations in metabolic functioning, uterine bleeding, and impaired mobility are the major diagnostic categories for breastfeeding women.

KEY CONCEPTS

Asthma - About one percent of pregnant women have asthma. Aerosal inhaled corticosteriods lessen the amont of drug transferred into breastmilk. If the mother is taking theophylline, monitor the infant for irritability.

Cystic fibrosis - A dysfunction of the exocrine glands. Mother with cystric fibrosis may breastfeed with close nutritional monitoring.

Diabetes - An illness involving impaired carbohydrate metabolism caused by insufficient insulin. Breastfeeding lowers blood glucose levels and helps the mother with diabetes feel normal following a high risk pregnancy.

Dysfunctional uterine bleeding - Several different factors cause abnormal, excessive uterine bleeding. The mother should receive immediate medical intervention, usually Methergine and possibly curettage of the uterine linning.

Hyperthyroidism - An excess of thyroid hormone. Breastfeeding is not affected. Propylthiouracil is the treatment of choice during lactation.

Hypothyroidism - Thyroid deficiency can reduce milk volume. Replacement therapy of thyroid extract may increase the milk supply in affected women.

Induced lactation - Induced lactation (usually practiced when a mother adopts an infant) in non-postpartum women is a slow process. Induced lactation/relactation requires close monitoring by a qualified lactation consultant.

Infections - Most infections in healthy childbearing women are self-limiting. In many cases, the infant receives valuable antibodies against the infection in the mother's milk. Antibiotics are almost always compatible with breastfeeding. See p. 357 in the text for information regarding maternal chickenpox.

Maternal nutrition - Maternal nutrition substantially affects breastmilk composition and volume only when the mother is severely malnourished. Breastfeeding women tend to lose more weight after birth than their bottle-feeding counterparts.

Maternal smoking - Maternal smoking aggravates infant allergies and increases respiratory illness. Mothers addicted to nicotine should smoke outside and after (not before) feedings to reduce the effect of secondhand smoke on their baby.

Multiple sclerosis - A progressive degenerative neurologic disorder. Women with multiple sclerosis may breastfeed, except in the case of severe illness from an exacerbation of the disease.

Pituitary dysfunction - With appropriate medical treatment, breastfeeding should not be restricted in women with prolactinomas or other forms of pituitary dysfunction.

Postpartum depression - Most women experience a transient depression following birth. True postpartum depression occurs in about 20 percent of women in the USA. Postpartum psychosis is rare. A medication compatible with breastfeeding should be selected, family support provided, and the mother and baby kept together.

Radioisotope studies - Diagnostic studies using radioactive isotopes usually require that breastfeeding be interrupted until nearly all radioactivity is excreted. Consult guidelines on pp. 370-373 of the text for specific radioisotopes.

Relactation - Restimulating lactation after it has ceased in a postpartum woman. The shorter the period since birth, the greater the chance of success. Relactation requires anticipatory guidance and intensive assistance from a qualified lactation consultant.

Rheumatoid arthritis - A chronic inflammatory auto-immune disorder. The symptoms usually go into remission during pregnancy and relapse postpartum. A client advocate may be needed to select medications compatible with breastfeeding.

Seizure disorder - Women with a seizure disorder may breastfeed as any other mother would. Commonly prescribed medications for seizure disorders are usually compatible with breastfeeding.

READINGS FOR FURTHER REFERENCE

Coates MM, Riordan J: (1992) Breastfeeding during maternal or infant illness. *In Clin Iss Perinat Wom Health Nurs* 3: 683-94.

Conine TA, Carty, E. and Safarik PM 1988: *Aids and Adaptation for Parents with Physical or Sensory Disabilities.* Vancouver, B.C., School of Rehabilitative Medicine, University of British Columbia, Canada, pp. 67-71. Order from the University.

May, KA, Mahlmeister, LR: *Maternal and Neonatal Nursing*, 3rd ed. Philadelphia: JB Lippincott, 1994; see esp. Chapters 27, 29, and 34.

La Leche League, International
Booklets and Packets:
"The diabetic mother and breastfeeding" (No. 17), $0.95
"Nutrition and breastfeeding" (No. 159), $.60

New Beginnings and *Leaven,* published by LLLI, are rich sources of cases and information about health problems of breastfeeding women. Contact your local La Leche League for copies. They are not usually found in public libraries or on electronic data bases.

LEARNING ACTIVITIES

1. Prepare a list of maternal health problems and benefits that relate to breastfeeding (see TR 13-1). (I)

2. Have your students select one maternal health problem and write a paper about it with appropriate references and documentation. Include an interview an individual who has had personal experience with this problem either as a breastfeeding mother or as a health care provider. (S)

3. Present a case report of one maternal health problem that relates to breastfeeding. Include laboratory data, medications and interventions, family responses and outcomes. (S)

4. Present crisis intervention concepts and techniques to the class. Discuss how crisis interventions could be used to assist lactating mothers who suddenly experience a health crisis. (I,S)

5. Describe each of the maternal health problems listed in this chapter. In each case, identify key signs and symptoms and note the implications of the health problem for: (I,S)
   a. breastfeeding initiation
   b. unimpaired lactation
   c. continued breastfeeding

6. What is induced lactation and when might it be considered an appropriate option? (I,S)

7. What is relactation? How is it similar to, different from, induced lactation? (I,S)

8. Refer to TR 13-2 when discussing each of the elements listed and their importance when considering relactation or induced lactation. (I, S)

9. Review and discuss the incidence and prevalence of postpartum depression. In what way(s) are each of the elements listed in TR13-3 related to: (I,S)
   a. new parenthood?
   b. breastfeeding?
   c. hormone changes?
   d. stress?

10. How might breastfeeding reduce/increase the likelihood/severity of postpartum depression? How is separation of mother and infant implicated in the frequency of postpartum depression? (I)

11. In what way(s) do the three types of postpartum depression (refer to TR 13-4) relate to how new mothers are managed? (I)

12. Invite a clinical pharmacist to discuss the pros and cons of use of each of the medications listed in TR 13-5 and 13-6 by the breastfeeding mother with postpartum depression. (I)

13. Discuss when radiation therapy is necessary and how it might be used during lactation (see TR 13-7). (I)

CHAPTER 14

Breast-Related Problems

Breastfeeding counseling often involves breast related problems.This chapter reviews specific breast problems that relate to breastfeeding and discusses how health professionals can help mothers to overcome them. Many breast problems during lactation result from lack of knowledge; others are the result of medical technology—candidiasis is a case in point. Client advocacy and education is a thread that runs throughout this chapter.

KEY CONCEPTS

Breast augmentation - A surgical implant to enlarge breasts. The effect of augmentation on subsequent ability to lactate is individual and not predictible.

Breast cancer - Very rare in lactating women; however, any suspicious lump in the breast should be evaluated by a experienced surgeon. Breastfeeding protects against premenopausal breast cancer.

Breast reduction - Surgical removal of fatty tissue in the breast to reduce breast size. Breastfeeding may be possible with the pedicle technique, but is less likely with the free-nipple/areola technique.

Candidiasis - A yeast infection involving the breast tissue and/or the infant's oral cavity. Symptoms include pain and inflammatory process on the breast skin. Interventions include medications (clotrimazole, nystatin, miconazole, diflucan) used on affected area. The infant (oral cavity and diaper/nappy area) should also be assessed and treated prophylatically.

Fibrocystic breast disease - Benign breast cysts. Fibrocystic changes are common in women of childbearing age and constitute from 50% to 75% of all breast biopsies. A needle aspiration and laboratory study confirm the diagnosis.

Inverted nipples - True inversion is uncommon, but can be a barrier to breastfeeding. Exercising the nipple just before latch on is the most effective intervention for inversion. Breast shells and Hoffman exercises are, for the most part, ineffective.

Mastitis - A local infection of the breast. Symptoms include fatigue, tenderness, muscular aching, and fever. Mastitis usually involves staphylococcus and is self-limiting unless it is a streptococcus infection, which is more serious.

Mastoplexy - "Breastlift;" it does not affect the ability to breastfeed.

Plugged ducts - Non-communication between the ducts and the nipple opening caused by pathologic changes causing the "plug." Symptoms are tenderness, redness , lumpiness, or a tiny white plug seen at the nipple opening. Interventions include moist heat, massage, soaking the affected breast, and changing feeding positions.

READING FOR FURTHER REFERENCE

Baumslag, M, Michels, DL: *A Woman's Guide to Yeast Infection.* New York: Pocket Books, 1992.

Love, SM: *Dr. Susan Love's Breast Book*, Rev. Ed. Reading, MA: Addison-Wesley Publishing Co., Inc., 1995.

LEARNING ACTIVITIES

1. Discuss breast surgery and its implications for breastfeeding. Refer to TR 14-2, 14-3, 14-4 in your discussion. (I,S)

2. Invite five women to present their story to the class. Each woman has had one or more of the following breast surgeries: (I)
   a. breast augmentation
   b. breast reduction
   c. mastopexy
   d. removal of a breast cyst or benign tumor
   e. breast reconstruction following accident or illness

   In each case, ask the woman to identify:
      1) *when* the surgery was done
      2) *why* it was done
      3) whether it occurred before or after her decision to have children
      4) whether it occurred before or after her decision to breastfeed
      5) any effects on breastfeeding of the surgery; and her feelings about that.

3. Distinguish between a plugged duct and mastitis (refer to TR 14-1, 14-5). (I, S)

4. Discuss candidiasis. Compare treatments, course of treatment, and their likely effectiveness. In what order might multiple treatments be suggested? why? (I,S)

5. Develop a clinical care path for a breastfeeding woman who has discovered a firm lump in one of her breasts. (S)

6. Ask the students to review each of the items on TR 14-6, 14-7 and discuss the implications of each item for: (S)
   a. continued breastfeeding
   b. resolution of the problem
   c. likely continuation of the problem

7. Invite an oncologist to class to distinguish bewteen different kinds of breast cancer, when they are likely to occur, how they are identified, and how they can be distinguished from other more commonly-occurring experiences during lactation. (I)

8. Arrange a home visit to a breastfeeding mother and infant through a community health agency. Discuss any breast-related problems the mother may have postpartum, home remedies used and the sources she went to for information about the problem. (S)

9. Develop a specific research question from the chapter content on breast-related problems and a method of collecting data to answer the question. (S)

CHAPTER 15

Maternal Employment and Breastfeeding

This chapter reviews the history of maternal employment during the childbearing years and examines how such employment affects breastfeeding initiation and duration in developed countries, with primary focus on the United States. Ways in which to assist employed women to continue to breastfeed are discussed.

KEY CONCEPTS

1. **Bottle-feeding** - a technique of feeding from a receptable topped by a rubber or silicone teat designed to enable a suckling infant to obtain fluid nutriment. The technique used by a baby to obtain fluid from a bottle requires different activity than that employed when suckling the mother's breast. As a result, bottle-feeding has been implicated in problems manifested when breastfeeding is attempted after bottle-feeding has been initiated.

2. **Breast pumping** - usually the term referred to when a mechanical pump—whether it is hand-operated, battery- or electric-powered—is used to obtain milk from the breast in the absence of, or in addition to, suckling by the baby. Breast pumps vary in their efficiency and comfort; therefore, mothers depending on such devices to regularly obtain milk for their babies are well advised to select carefully the pump that works best for them. This is particularly true when long-term use is contemplated.

3. **Cup-feeding** - a technique for feeding an infant that does not require sucking, but rather depends on a sipping or lapping action. Cup-feeding can be used from birth, with preterm as well as term infants, and offers an alternative to bottle-feeding when the risks it represents exceed the benefits it is assumed to confer.

4. **Day-care** - a term referring to care given to children by persons other than the mother. In most cases, daycare usually implies care at a site not in the baby's home. It also infers group care insofar as more than one child usually is cared for by the same individual or team of caregivers.

5. **Expressing milk** - the term used to refer to obtaining milk by hand, with or without the use of a mechanical device such as a breast pump. Hand expression is a learned skill and thus takes time in which to gain proficiency. It is, however, less expensive than breast pumping and the equipment needed (breast and hand) is always available. The efficiency with which an individual expresses her milk is dependent, for the most part, on what she has been taught, and her interest in becoming skilled in its implementation.

6. **Fatigue** - with regard to maternal experiences, one of the characteristics of motherhood. With regard to employed motherhood, one of the most frequent complaints of busy mothers, regardless of how they feed their babies.

7. **Maternity leave** - a time period, varying by country as well as state/provincial and/or local laws that provides a new mother with time off from her regular paid employment in order to meet the needs of her new infant. In some cases, such leave lasts a few weeks, in other settings, several months. In the United States, such leave is unpaid and is guaranteed only by federal law affecting companies with 50

or more employees; thus it affects only a small minority of companies. As of 1994, the Republic of South Africa is the only industrialized country with no federally mandated maternity leave, paid or unpaid.

8. **Milk storage** - a term referring to the collection of milk for later use by the mother's own infant, usually in her absence. Stor-age mechanisms may include refrigeration and/or freezing, although raw fresh milk also may be collected and stored for later use. How and in what kind of container such milk is stored can influence how easily it can be used.

9. **Prenatal Planning** - the planning that occurs during a woman's pregnancy and which she expects to carry out after the baby's birth. With regard to breastfeeding in general and to combining breastfeeding with paid employment in particular, planning that anticipates needs often contributes to a more pleasant and problem-free experience.

10. **"Reverse Cycle Nursing"** - a term referring to the breastfeeding pattern exhibited by many babies younger than six months of age whose mothers are employed and separated from them during the day. In such a circumstance, frequent feeds are more likely to occur during those times when the mother is available, with sleep periods occurring during those hours when other babies might be breastfeeding. Understanding such patterns and recognizing them as a means by which maternal-infant closeness can be enhanced is likely to assist a mother whose friends, relatives, and advisors are unacquainted with such behavior and whose subsequent advice might not be entirely appropriate.

11. **Social Support** - the assistance provided by others whose relationship with the employed breastfeeding mother renders their advice or recommendations particularly important. In many cases, her spouse and other relatives form the primary, most continuous source of support for the breastfeeding mother. Other persons who might become members of this support system include health care providers, other employees, other breast-feeding mothers, and especially other employed breastfeeding mothers.

12. **Spoon-feeding** - A method of feeding a baby that uses a spoon rather than a cup, a bottle, or direct breastfeeding. Both solid and semi-solid foods and fluids can be given by spoon. When semi-solid or solid foods are offered, this technique is most appropriately taught after the extrusion reflex is extinguished, usually at about four months of age or later.

13. **The "5-15-5" rule** - Five minutes of expressing milk is usually sufficient to reduce uncomfortable fullness and occurs at mid-morning or mid-afternoon breaks; 15 minutes refers to expressing to store milk, even if the mother does not need that much time to do so and occurs at a meal break. This rule is most appropriately applied when the mother has recently returned to work and/or before her baby's fourth month of life. Later return to work when infant feeding patterns are less frequent may not require application of the "5-15-5" rule.

LEARNING ACTIVITIES

1. Describe the different ways in which bottle-feeding might be combined with breastfeeding when the mother is employed outside the home. Refer to TR 15-1 and 15-2 when asddressing the issue. (I)

2. Using the continuum of options (see TR 15-3), invite mothers representing each place on the continuum to speak to the class about what they chose, why they chose it, when they returned to work and how their choice influenced their lactation course and breastfeeding duration. (I)

3. Review the elements in TR 15-2 regarding questions a mother should ask when selecting a breast pump. Explain how each element can affect a mother's breast pumping regimen and breastfeeding experience after she returns to work. (I)

4. Invite at least three mothers to present a panel of breast pumping experiences to the class. Select mothers who have each used a different kind of breast pump. (I)

5. Explain cup-feeding and how it differs from breastfeeding or bottle-feeding. (I)

6. Have a mother show the class how she cup-feeds her infant. If cup-feeding is practiced in a local hospital, ask a nurse to show how she cup-feeds a newborn (**NB**: The mother's written permission must be obtained prior to such a demonstration.) (I)

7. Review each of the barriers (see TR 15-4) to combining breastfeeding and employment outside the home. Review how each might be reduced or eliminated as a factor influencing women (I)
   a. not to work outside the home when they have small children
   b. not to breastfeed when employed outside the home.

8. Ask your students to visit two examples of each of the following kinds of day-care facilities: (S)
   a. private home with only their own children cared for there;
   b. private home with fewer than five children —not from that home;
   c. home with more than five unrelated children; and,
   d. day care facility with more than 10 children.
   For each facility, have the students ask:
      1) what is the daily, weekly, monthly fee?
      2) how was the caregiver identified?
      3) is the home/facility licensed? If so, by whom? If not, why not?
      4) what is the difference between a licensed and an unlicensed facility in this city, county or parish, state or province?
      5) how familiar with a breastfeeding baby is the caregiver?
      6) how many breastfeeding babies in the past two years has the facility cared for?
      7) how long was each baby breastfed?
      8) is there a place for mothers to breastfeed on site?
      9) how familiar with handling breastmilk is the staff?
      10) what problems specific to breastfeeding babies have they encountered?
      11) how do the answers to 10) above reflect a bottle-feeding society?

9. Ask a panel of four mothers to explain why they chose their day care facility. Each should have used one of the following sites: (I)
   a. her own home with the substitute caretaker coming to the home;
   b. a private home in the neighborhood
   c. a relative
   d. a day care facility near the home
   e. a day care facility at or near the mother's work

10. Review day care options (see TR 15-6) and provide information on the availability of each in the local community. (I)

11. Contact one or more local businesses and ask them to send a representative to explain to the class why they have chosen to provide on-site daycare for their employees. If no such businesses offer such a service, ask them why they do not. In each case, inquire how their service (or lack of same) affects their breastfeeding employees, their ability to retain women workers. (I)

12. Invite two or more mothers to demonstrate hand-expression. Ask each to explain: (I)
    a. *why* they chose this method of obtaining milk
    b. *who*, if anyone, taught them hand expression
    c. *how long* they practiced before getting good at it
    d. *what* they would tell other mothers about it
    e. *how long* they were able to supply all of the baby's milk needs during their absence

13. Discuss three reasons for expressing milk and explain how each is affected by: (I,S)
    a. timing of the mother's return to work
    b. number of hours she works each day

14. Review how loss of sleep can affect daytime functioning in adults. What factors regarding breastfeeding can assist a mother to obtain needed rest in order to cope with shorter periods than previous amounts of uninterrupted night sleep? (I)

15. Invite an expert in postpartum depression to the class to discuss the effect of sleep deprivation on new parents and its possible relationship to depressive episodes. How does breastfeeding affect postpartum depression? How does postpartum depression affect breastfeeding? (I)

16. Invite representatives of up to five businesses (at least one of which is a health care institution) in your community to explain their policy regarding maternity leave: its length, paid or unpaid, whether it can be combined with accrued vacation time to make it longer, whether paternal leave is also available, and whether mothers wishing to return parttime may do so. Are babies allowed at the worksite? May breastfeeding babies come in to be breastfed? [**NB**: Be sure to include at least two businesses with fewer than 50 employees.] (I)

17. Invite five fathers of young babies to share their early experiences with parenthood with the class. Ask them to present the father's perspective regarding the maternity leave available and/or used by their mates.
    a. How did this leave, if any, affect the fathers?
    b. Did the fathers take similar leave? If so, why? If not, why not?
    c. How did the fathers feel about returning to work for the first time after ~~the~~ baby's birth? (I)

18. Review general guidelines for storing human milk. Give rationales for each. Provide examples when the mother might choose to provide... for those feedings when she is not present to breastfeed. (I)
    a. fresh milk
    b. refrigerated milk
    c. lightly frozen milk
    d. deeply frozen milk

19. Ask a panel of employed breastfeeding mothers to explain how they stored their milk, why they did so in that manner, problems they encountered, from whom—if anyone—they sought advice about milk storage, and what they would recommend to others. (I)

20. Review ways in which a pregnant mother might make plans for breastfeeding after returning to paid work. Discuss the pros and cons of such planning. (I)

21. Invite two or more parent educators to review for the class what they recommend to pregnant women regarding breastfeeding, and breastfeeding and working. After their presentation, ask the class to critique the completeness and appropriateness of their recommendations. (S)

22. Explain what is meant by reverse cycle nursing. (I)

23. Review the five different types of social support (see TR 15-5). Identify by occupation and by relation to the mother who these people might be. (I,S)

24. Ask a panel of mothers to identify *who* served in each of the five roles of social support for her. Have these persons changed since her baby's birth? Have her needs changed over time so that one person is now more important than someone else? If so, in what way(s)? who? (I)

25. Invite 5 health care workers (representing different occupations, if possible) to share panel duties as each explains *how* they combined new parenthood and breastfeeding with employment, the problems they encountered, whether and/or how they were resolved, and the impact of their personal experience on what they advise their patients. (I)

26. Invite two mothers to class to demonstrate spoon-feeding liquids and solid or semi-solid food to this infant. Ask each mother to describe when they began doing so and why. (I)

27. Examine the "5-15-5 rule" as a theoretical construct. Identify the pros and cons of such a recommendation. (I,S)

28. Ask 5 mothers to explain how often they expressed/pumped their breasts over time. How long did they do so, how long for each pattern of expressing/pumping (3x, 2x, 1x/day, and so on) and what factors contributed to their decisions in changing patterns? (I)

CHAPTER 16

Fertility, Sexuality, and Contraception During Lactation

This chapter examines fertility, sexuality and contraception and how each influences and is affected by the lactation course. Family planning issues and how they relate to breastfeeding also are discussed.

KEY CONCEPTS

1. **Amenorrhea** - A period during which fertility is not possible. Lactation amenorrhea refers to that period when lactation prevents conception.

2. **Contraception** - actions taken to prevent conception during potentially fertile periods in presumably fertile sex partners. Contraception may include abstinence, barrier methods, non-hormonal methods, hormonal methods, and/or sterilization.

3. **Double protection** - the period between the time when family planning begins before amenorrhea ends, thereby seeking to prevent conception before its likelihood of occurrence is substantial.

4. **Family planning** - techniques by which sex partners seek to control the number and spacing of children they wish to conceive and rear.

5. **Fertility** - the ability to conceive; this capability will be influenced by a variety of factors, including the degree to which suppressing effects, such as breastfeeding, are practiced.

6. **Intercourse** - the act of sexual expression that can result in conception.

7. **Libido** - sexual desire or drive. Libido can be inhibited or enhanced by lactation, situational factors, pregnancy, and birth, for both sex partners.

8. **Ovulation patterns** - the pattern pertaining to release of an egg by the woman. The frequency of ovulation during the childbearing years can be reduced by several factors, including lactation.

9. **Sexuality** - the expression of one's gender identity. Such expression may be identified as heterosexuality or homosexuality.

10. **Supplemental feeding** - those feedings offered to infants or young children in addition to, or in replacement of, breastfeeding. Supplemental feeding can reduce the suppressing effect of lactation on amenorrhea and ovulation.

LEARNING ACTIVITIES

1. Review the relationship between fertility, sexuality, contraception, and lactation (see TR 16-1). (I)

2. Describe the usual menstrual cycle and how it relates hormonally to the patterns immediately post-delivery and through the lactation course (see TR 16-4). Identify when amenorrhea occurs and how it is affected by lactation. (I)

3. Review different methods of contraception (see p. 447). Identify risks and benefits of each method related to use and protection during lactation. (I)

4. Have a panel of women describe their contraceptive patterns during the first five years of their life with their sex partner. Ask the students to note differences and similarities between the women's experiences. Have them note when/if contraceptive failure occurred and how this was resolved. (S)

5. Describe and discuss the implications of "double protection," (See TR 16-3; p.448) for populations in developed countries, developing countries. (I,S)

6. Invite a panel of family planning experts to the class. Each will mention the following: (I)
   a. age of the women seeking family planning information/methods;
   b. marital status of the women seeking family planning information/methods;
   c. methods of family planning the women use
   d. problems expressed

7. Ask the students to examine Table 16-1 of the text (p. 445) and to explain the differences in frequency of intercourse following birth of a baby in three cities. Ask them to explain these differences. (S)

8. Define libido and how each of five categories of factors can influence libido during lactation and at other times (see TR 16-2). (I)

9. Invite a panel of mothers to come to class and discuss their own ovulation patterns over time (these mothers should have two or more children in order to compare differences between children and their own related changes in fertility over time). Students should be prepared to ask questions relating to factors that may have influenced timing of the women's ovulation and subsequent fertility. (S)

10. Describe different expressions of sexuality and how they relate to lactation. (I)

11. Explain how supplemental feeding can influence lactation and fertility or subfertility. (I)

CHAPTER 17

Child Health

Breastfeeding is health promotion and health begins at birth. This chapter begins with an overview of normal growth and development and reviews prominent thories of child development. including attachment and bonding. Studies of cognitive and social development between breastfed and bottle-fed infants are reviewed.

KEY CONCEPTS

1. **Arousal** - A continuum of levels of consciousness of the infant.

2. **Attachment** - The human equivalent of imprinting by the infant to the mother and later to other significant individuals. Attachment is progressive and takes place over time though initimate, cue-based interactions.

3. **Communication** - Children acquire language communication in a consistent sequence. Crying is a form of communication that the infant needs something—either attention or food or both.

4. **Dental health** - Breastfed infants have less dental disease and malocclusion.

5. **Immunization** - One means by which the recipient is protected against certain diseases. Breastfed infants receive the same schedule of immunizations as infants not breastfed, but respond with higher titer levels than non-breastfed infants receiving the same immunizations.

6. **Nature vs. nurture** - The continuing controversy about which factor is more important: nature (genes, heredity) or nurture (parenting and social development).

7. **Obesity** - Breastfeeding has a far weaker effect on subsequent obesity of the child than genetic, racial, and socioeconomic factors.

8. **Reflexes** - Highly developed at birth and designed to enhance survival. Rooting, suckling, swallowing, and gagging are reflexes that facilitate breastfeeding.

9. **Senses**- Highly developed at birth except for vision. Through their senses, infants can discriminate among sound, heat, pleasure, and pain.

10. **Separation** - Anxiety or loud protest when the mother or significant caretaker leaves the infant. Begins around six months and ends soon after the second year birthday.

11. **Social development** - Process of developing language and relating to persons in the environment in a meaningful, yet individual way.

12. **Stranger distress** - Loud protest upon the approach of a stranger even when the mother or significant caretaker is present.

13. **Temperament** - Infants have individual personality characteristics or temperament "styles" that affect breastfeedings and nurturing needs.

14. **Weaning** - Slow, gradual introduction of other foods into the infant's diet. Baby-led weaning is recommended as optimal for child nurturing.

READINGS FOR FURTHER REFERENCE

Ainsworth, MDS, et al.: *Patterns of Attachment.* Hillsdale, NJ: Lawrence Erlbaum Associates, Inc., 1978.

Bowlby, JL: *Attachment and Loss: Vol. 1, Separation.* NY: Basic Books, Inc., 1973.

Rubin R: Attainment of the maternal role, I. Processess. II. Models and referrants, *Nurs Res* 16:237, 342, 1967.

Whaley, LF, Wong, DL: *Nursing Care of Infants and Children*, 5th ed. St. Louis, MO: C.V. Mosby, 1995.

LEARNING ACTIVITIES

1. Describe psychological/psychosocial attachment and how it relates to infant health. How is secure attachment related to the ability to separate? (I)

2. Review the stages of communication from birth through the ability to write. How does breastfeeding as an infant experience relate to infant and young child communication? (I)

3. In what way(s) is breastfeeding related to early and later dental health? (S)

4. Discuss "nature vs. nurture" and how each contributes to the growth and development of a child. (I, S)

5. How is obesity determined? In what way is breastfeeding related to obesity in infants? (I,S)

6. Review infant reflexes and how they relate to breastfeeding. (I)

7. Review the five senses and how infants and young children use each to explore their world. (I, S)

8. Explain stranger distress. Review different ways in which children respond to strangers and the implications of such reactions on the intensity/nature of their attachment to a parent. (I)

9. Describe each of the following forms of weaning: abrupt, gradual, planned (refer to TR 2-2). In each case, when is it likely to occur, and what effect (if any) might it have on a) the lactating mother; b) the breastfeeding baby/young child? (I,S)

10. Invite four directors of day care centers to the class. Ask them to describe how their facility accommodates breastfeeding babies and the differences they have observed, if any, between breastfeeding and non-breastfeeding infants in their care. (I)

11. Ask your students to go to the grocery store. (S)
    a. What different kinds of mixed foods for infants and young children are available?
    b. How old are the infants pictured in the ad copy/food container?
    c. When do the instructions for use recommend using the product?
    d. If there is a difference between b) and c) above, how do you explain that difference?
    e. Which of these mixed foods is essential to normal growth and development?
    f. Read the labels. What ingredients might one question as non-essential to human growth/development?
    g. What is the nutritional value of these foods? What might the infant/young child gain from use of these foods at 1 month, 3 months, 6 months, 9 months, 12 months?
    h. What alternatives to these foods are available to
        1) low-income mothers?
        2) mothers without microwave ovens?
        3) mothers working outside the home?

12. (See TR 17-1). Discuss how and why artificial feeding represents such an increased risk for each of the conditions listed.

CHAPTER 18

The Ill Breastfeeding Baby

This chapter describes health problems of infants and children in relation to breastfeeding. Health-care workers must know when and how to effectively help the mother of an ill child without unnecessarily disrupting breastfeeding.

KEY CONCEPTS

1. **Allergies** - An abnormal response to foods, drugs or inhalants. Symptoms in infants include diarrhea, eczema, vomiting, and colic. Cow's milk protein is a common allergen of infants.

2. **Celiac Disease** - Poor absorption of fat in the intestinal mucosa; caused by sensitivity to gluten in wheat, rye, oats, and barley. The infant's stools are frothy and foul smelling. Exclusive breastfeeding delays and ameliorates the onset of the disease.

3. **Choanal atresia** - Narrowing of the posterior nares prevent the infant from breathing normally. Reconstructive surgery is done early. The infant usually can breastfeed if careful attention is paid to the airway; breastmilk also may given through NG tube.

4. **Cleft lip/palate** - Congenital malformation with incomplete fusing of the central processes around lip and palate. Reconstructive surgery occurs early. Breast-feeding is possible and encouraged.

5. **Congenital heart defect** - May not be recognized after birth. The infant tires easily at the breast and may fail to gain adequate weight. Surgery may be indicated. Breastfeeding is encouraged as a protection against infections. Upright positioning and short feedings make it easier for the infant to breastfeed.

6. **Congenital hypothyroidism** - Congenital lack of thyroid secretion; occurs in1:5000 birth. Breastmilk contains small quantities of thyroid hormones and may provide minimal protection in early weeks. The afflicted child will need lifelong thyroid replacement.

7. **Cystic fibrosis** - A congenital disease in which the glands produce abnormally thick and sticky secretions; occurs in 1:2000 births. Intestinal obstruction can occur and respiratory infections are common. Breastfeeding is encouraged as the lipase in breastmilk is protective against symptoms.

8. **Down syndrome** - A congenital condition characterized by epicanthal folds, broad hand, simian crease, flattened forehead, hypotonicity, increased risk of upper respiratory infections, and a range of mental retardation from mild to profound. Breastfeeding is encouraged. Hypotonicity may require special handling during feedings.

9. **Esophageal reflux** - Self-limiting persistent nonprojectile vomiting because of laxity of the lower eso-phageal muscles. This problem is more pronounced in artificially-fed infants.

10. **Gastrointestinal infection** - Viral or bacterial invasion of the GI tract. Dehydration from vomiting and diarrhea is the greatest danger. Breastfed infants are half as likely as artificially-fed infants to develop GI infection.

11. **Hydrocephalus** - Accumulation of fluid in the

intracranial cavity caused by excess cerebrospinal fluid. Surgery to bypass the obstruction is done early. Breastfeeding is often possible and encouraged.

11. **Hypoglycemia** - Blood glucose reaches lowest its level between one and two hours after birth and gradually rises. Symptoms are tremors, jitteriness, lethargy, and a weak or high-pitched cry. Definition of "normal" blood glucose values of neonates varies among hospitals. If 30% or below in the first 24 hours is used, incidence rates are around 7%.

12. **Imperforate anus** - Blind rectal pouch that requires surgical correction. Breastfeeding is especially encouraged to protect the infant from secondary infection.

13. **Inborn error of metabolism** - A congenital chromosomal "error" of metabolism; PKU is an example. Breastfeeding is encouraged because breastmilk contains low levels of phenylalanine; low-phenylalanine formula may be used as supplement. Galactosemia, another inborn error of metabolism, is one of the few cases where the infant cannot breastfeed.

14. **"Magic milk" syndrome** - A part of grieving over a chronically ill child, parents perceive breastmilk as having "magical" properties that will heal their baby.

15. **Meningitis\Myelomeningocele** - Acute inflammation of meninges caused by viral or bacterial pathogen. Nausea, vomiting and neurological signs result. Breastmilk is protective against bacterial meningitis.

16. **Otitis media** - Inflammation of the middle ear. Prevalent in children; usually caused by *H. Influenzae* and treated with amoxicillin, a penicillinase-resistant antibiotic. Breastfeeding helps protect the child against ear infections.

17. **Pyloric stenosis** - Severe projectile vomiting a few weeks after birth presumably from hypertrophy of the pyloric sphincter. Surgery corrects the problem. This seldom occurs in the breastfed infant.

18. **Respiratory infection** - Respiratory syncytial virus (RSV) is a common respiratory infection in infants. Breastmilk is protective against viral respiratory disease.

19. **Sudden Infant Death Syndrome (SIDS)** - Occurs 1:1000 births. Called "crib death" or "cot death;" refers to sudden death without warning. Lack of breastfeeding is risk factor for SIDS.

20. **Tracheoesophageal fistula** - Abnormal opening between the trachea and esophagus; occurs in about 1:3000 births. Colostrum, a physiologic fluid, is much less irritating to the lungs if aspirated than water, glucose water, or artificial infant milks.

READINGS FOR FURTHER REFERENCE

Bets, CL, Hunsberger, M, Wright, S: *Nursing Care of Children, 2nd ed.* Philadelphia: W.B. Saunders Company, 1994.

The Compassionate Friends: *When a Baby Dies.* Centering Corporation, 1531 N. Saddle Creed Rd, Omaha, NE 68104 USA.

McFadden, EA: *Case Studies in the Nursing of Children and Families.* Baltimore, MD: Williams and Wilkins, 1989.

LEARNING ACTIVITIES

1. What is the infant mortality rate in different countries worldwide? (Include the elements shown in TR 18-2 in your discussion of the impact of infant loss on the surviving family members. (Select 5 developed, and 5 developing countries). What do their respective IM rates tell you about their society? (I)

2. Review infant illness (see TR 18-1) and examine how breastfeeding can assist the baby and the family during the period of illness. (I,S)

3. Distinguish between neonatal (1-28 days) and postneonatal (28-364 days) mortality. For each mortality period, how might the absence of breastfeeding be reflected? (HINT: what diseases/ problems are most likely to occur neonatally or postneonatally? Why? (I,S)

4. Describe neurological dysfunction, how it is likely to be manifested and in what ways it is related to early and later feeding behavior (see TR 18-4). (I,S)

5. Invite five mothers to the class. Each mother will have give birth to a baby with one of the following conditions (I):
   a. hydrocephalus
   b. cleft lip
   c. cleft palate
   d. cystic fibrosis
   e. congenital heart defect (see TR 18-3)
   f. Down syndrome

   Ask each mother to describe how breastfeeding has been affected, if at all, by her baby's condition. Ask each mother to describe how her baby's health has been affected as a result of the condition by breastfeeding.

6. Invite a pediatric plastic surgeon to class. Ask her/him to describe how a cleft lip is repaired and how breastfeeding can be continued throughout the recuperative period and beyond. (I)

7. Review how allergies manifest themselves and what a mother can do to reduce their likelihood of occurrence (or effect once they occur) in the infant/young child. (I)

8. Discuss how breastfeeding can normalize a life situation when a baby is born with a congenital defect/ condition. (I, S)

9. Review the literature on otitis media. In a paper, identify differences in occurrence, treatment, severity, and cost by how infants are fed. (S)

CHAPTER 19

Slow Weight Gain and Failure to Thrive

This chapter examines factors that may contribute to slow weight gain in the healthy breastfeeding baby, contrasting these elements with those that may contribute to nutritional failure to thrive. Distinguishing between maternal factors and infant factors relating to failure to gain also are discussed.

KEY CONCEPTS

1. **Disorganized Suckling** - A pattern of suckling that is ineffective in obtaining milk from the breast through stimulation of the maternal milk ejection reflex. Very often, the infant will suckle with his eyes closed throughout the feed, will suckle and swallow infrequently followed by a fluttering action of the chin, will exhibit a suckle described by the mother as very soft, weak, or not strong, or that hurts her. Often, the mother does not report observing or hearing much swallowing. Such a pattern of suckling precedes a diagnosis of nutritional failure to thrive.

2. **Failure to Thrive** - A diagnosis applied to infants whose weight, when plotted on a standardized growth chart, drops below the third percentile or two standard deviations below the mean for a particular age or height or both. Two other definitions also used is failure to regain birth weight by the third week of life or gaining an average of fewer than four ounces (114 cc) per week.

3. **Growth Charts** - Charts devised separately for boys and girls, which indicate expected rates of change in height (length), weight, and weight for height respectively over time. Most such tools were standardized when infant feeding patterns were considerably different than current patterns.

4. **Hypothyroidism** - One factor that needs to be ruled out in the mother as a cause of insufficient milk production. If the mother's thyroid level can be corrected, milk production may approach adequate levels in the absence of infant-related problems that might contribute to such an outcome. An infant with hypothyroidism also may have a poor suck, gain weight slowly, and stool infrequently. This condition needs to be ruled out or corrected if identified.

5. **Inadequate Caloric Intake** - Intake of calories insufficient to sustain growth as well as survival. Usually, the first indication of this insufficiency is failure to sustain weight gain, followed by a slowing of increases in height, and—lastly—head circumference.

6. **Insufficient Feedings** - Feedings that are not frequent enough, of sufficient duration or effectiveness to sustain appropriate growth as well as survival. Often, insufficient feedings are a result of inappropriate management in the hospital.

7. **Insufficient Glandular Tissue** - A maternal condition inferred from evaluation of both mother and infant in which the mother's response to breast and nipple stimulation is minimal or absent. In this case, the mother is unable to make sufficient milk because the amount of glandular tissue in the breasts is minimal. In many cases, mothers with this condition have assymetric breasts markedly different in both size and shape. The absence of sufficient tissue need not, however, preclude continued breastfeeding. With the use of supplemental milk offered at the breast, the mother and baby can continue to enjoy a breastfeeding relationship.

8. **Neurologic Dysfunction** - A problem for some infants which may be temporary or an indication of a neurologic problem of varying severity. This dysfunction is reflected in a pattern of poor suckling. In situations of hypertonia, increasing infant maturity often resolves the problem. In situations of hypotonia, gradually improving muscle tone may help, as well as the use of feeding tube devices designed to optomize milk transfer with minimal effort.

9. **Normal Growth** - The expected pattern of growth of term healthy infants which includes the following parameters: weight loss of 5-10% of birth weight followed by regaining same by the second week of life; doubling birth weight by five to six months of age, and tripling birth weight by one year; an increase in head circumference of 7.6 cm (3 inches) at one year. Variations occur; in particular, rate of gain is more rapid for breastfed babies in the first third of the first year and then slows more rapidly than the growth rate of artificially-fed infants.

10. **Positioning** - One obvious, but frequently overlooked, factor in evaluating causative variables underlying inadequate infant weight gain. Frequently, correction of poor positioning so that both mother and infant are comfortable and so that the infant need not expend excess energy in order to feed adequately may be all that is necessary to resolve a pattern of poor weight gain.

11. **Slow-Gaining** - A condition that may create cause for concern even though the baby remains within the normal range for infant growth. Such infants are both healthy and happy and often share a genetic predisposition with siblings and/or parents to this pattern of growth. Intervention is rarely necessary unless mismanagement has contributed to such slow weight gain.

12. **Supplementation Devices** - Tools designed to provide the baby with additional milk than he may be receiving directly from his mother in order to sustain appropriate growth. Such devices include cups, spoons, and feeding tube devices. Rarely, a bottle will be used; because such a tool maybe a contributing factor in poor suckling. Therefore, a bottle is not usually considered an appropriate tool for supplementation.

13. **Tongue-Tie** - Sometimes called ankyloglossia, a condition whereby the tongue is tethered too tightly to the floor of the mouth, the result of which is poor suckling and characteristic tenderness of the mother's nipples. With this condition, many infants are unable to move the tongue forward over the lower gum. In some infants, the condition resolves spontaneously after the baby's frenulum is stretched sufficiently to allow greater freedom of the tongue. In other cases, clipping of the lingual frenulum may be necessary to allow effective suckling.

READINGS FOR FURTHER REFERENCE

Daly, SEJ, Hartmann, PE: Infant demand and milk supply, Part 1: Infant demand and milk production in lactating women. *J Hum Lact* 11:21-26, 1995.

Daly, SEJ, Hartmann, PE: Infant demand and milk supply, Part 2: The Short-term control of milk synthesis in lactating women. *J Hum Lact* 11:27-37, 1995.

Dewey KG, Heinig MJ, Nommsen LA, et al: Breastfed infants are leaner than formula-fed infants at 1 year of age: the DARLING study. *Am J Clin Nutr* 57:140-45, 1993.

Dewey KG, Heinig MJ, Nommsen LA, et al: Growth of breast-fed and formula-fed infants from 0 to 18 months: the DARLING study. *Pediatrics* 89:1035-41, 1992.

Renfrew M, Fisher C, Arms S: *Bestfeeding: Getting Breastfeeding Right for You*. Berkeley, CA: Celestial Arts, 1990.

Journal of Human Lactation 6:, September (entire issue), 1990.

LEARNING ACTIVITIES

1. Explain and characterize disorganized suckling and how to recognize it (refer to TR 19-1). (Show the video by the Royal College of Midwives and ask the students to identify problematic aspects of suckling. After they do so, review the same segments again and point out other aspects of each breastfeeding encounter which the students may have missed). (I)

2. Invite a panel of four mothers whose babies were diagnosed with nutritional failure to thrive to share their experiences with the class. In each case, ask them to reply to the following questions: (I)
   a. how old was the baby when the diagnosis was made? by whom?
   b. how had baby breastfeed prior to that time?
   c. how did the mother feel when the diagnosis was made?
   d. was the mother referred to anyone to assist the baby to breastfeed better? who referred? to whom?
   e. what was the cost of care to improve the baby's suck?
   f. how long did it take to improve the baby's suck?
   g. did this mother feel it was worth it?
   h. what would she tell other mothers whose baby has a similar problem?

3. Review alternatives available to mothers when their breastfeeding baby has been diagnosed with FTT (nutritional)? (I)

4. Show current growth charts commonly used. Why are they provided by the commercial baby milk companies? Compare differences by infant gender. (I)

5. If new breastfeeding infant growth charts are now available, compare them to previously used growth charts for all infants regardless of infant feeding pattern. (I)

6. Define hypothyroidism. How is it manifested in new mothers? new infants? What is its effect on lactation? infant breastfeeding pattern? Provide recommended protocols for managing breastfeeding in a mother who has hypothyroidism; in an infant found to have hypothyroidism. (I)

7. Ask your students to interview a woman who has been diagnosed with hypothyroidism; hyperthyroidism.
   a. How did she feed her baby?
   b. What was the outcome—if breastfeeding?
   c. What was the effect of her condition on the lactation course? (S)

8. Explain inadequate caloric intake in infants by first explaining what is expected. Then review factors—management, infant-related, and maternal-related—that can contribute to this outcome (see TR 19-5). (I)

9. Explain insufficient feedings by discussing the following questions: (I,S)
   a. what is meant by the number of insufficient feedings for an infant?
   b. How might the likelihood of its occurrence be reduced through appropriate in-hospital management, later follow-up?
   c. Why is length of feeding as important as frequency?

10. Using a panel of breastfeeding mothers whose babies are at least six months, ask each to describe the frequency of their babies' feedings. Chart each pattern over time on an overhead and ask the class to come to a conclusion about the range of frequency that is normal, its relationship to infant weight gain (see references 1 and 2), and what could be shared with other mothers to reduce the likelihood of insufficiency of feedings. (I)

11. Invite two physicians (one obstetrician and one pediatrician) and one LC to explain how they determine whether "insufficient glandular tissue" is a possible explanation if a mother's baby is not gaining well. (I)

12. Explain what is meant by the term "insufficient glandular tissue." (I)

13. Examine TR 19-2 abd 19-3. Ask the students to extrapolate what they would expect of each mother-baby pair regarding: (S)
   a. labor medications on feeding frequency in the hospital
   b. management recommendations given in the hospital
   c. likelihood of supplementation (other fluids/foods); when given, if any
   d. likelihood of poor weight gain; adequate weight gain
   e. effect on expected duration of breastfeeding through six months of life

14. Now provide the following additional information. After initial discussion of question 13 above, consider the following experiences: (I)
   a. Baby 1 (first baby) was born without analgesia/anesthesia exposure in labor
   b. Baby 2 was considered small for gestational age at birth
   c. Baby 3 is the third child of a mother who bottle-fed her first two children
   d. Baby 4 was described by her mother as having "a very strong suck."
   e. Baby1 "acted sleepy" in the beginning, but "loves to nurse," according to his mother.
   f. Baby 2 is "very business-like."
   g. Baby 3 started receiving solids and one bottle a day at 10 weeks of age.
   h. Baby 4's mother returned to work at nine weeks postpartum.

   In each of the above cases, provide one piece of information and then ask the students if/why this information helps to explain frequency and/or duration of feeding episodes. Ask the students *which* baby characterizes *most* breastfeeding babies. [**ANSWER**: None; each is an individual with characteristics that *may* be shared by other babies.]

15. Invite 2-4 mothers who have been diagnosed with insufficient glandular tissue to explain: (I)
   a. when they received this diagnosis
   b. how they felt when they were told this
   c. how they then chose to feed their babies
   d. what they would tell other women about their experience

16. Review TR 19-4. Lead a class discussion of its significance and how it might be used to assist a new mother and baby. (S)

17. Explain how a baby might be determined to have a neurologic dysfucntion. Review situations that render this a temporary problem, a problem of gradually reducing significance, a continuing problem. (I)

18. Bring a panel of mothers with babies with a particular neurological problem (representing a range of severity) to the class. Ask them to explain how their baby's problem was discovered, how it is being managed, and its effect—if any—on the baby's feeding pattern. (I)

19. Review normal growth parameters and how they have been determined. Examine the references by Dewey; then lead a discussion pertaining to infant growth in different feeding groups, the appropriateness of new growth parameters for breastfeeding infants, their feasibility, whether they should be developed, and why. (I,S)

20. Invite a panel of pediatricians to debate the following question: "Growth parameters need to reflect whether a baby is breastfed or artificially fed. Current parameters are thus inadequate in assessing appropriate growth in the breastfed infant." Each side debating the question will present an initial argument for 5 minutes, with a 2-minute rebuttal statement. Thereafter, the class will vote their agreement with one or the other argument. (I)

21. Describe three variations of appropriate positioning. Explain and show with pictures (see Ref #11) how babies can be poorly positioned. (I)

22. "There are 152 positions to hold a baby and all of them are right." (Transparency #4). Show this transparency and ask the students what is important about the statement, and how they might use it when assisting a breastfeeding mother. (S)

23. Describe and discuss how a baby is determined to be gaining slowly and still be within the normal range. (Refer to TR 19-5.) (I)

24. Invite five mothers to describe their baby's growth in the first year of life (Two should be normal gainers, 2 slow gainers, 1 FTT). Do not label the mothers and ask them not to do so for their babies. Ask the students to identify which of the babies is a normal, but slow gaining baby, which one is considered to have failed to thrive, and which are considered appropriate normal gainers. (S)

25. Review the available devices in your community that can be used to supplement a baby's diet of breast-milk. In each case, review the risks and benefits of their use. (I)

26. Ask three mothers whose babies were diagnosed with nutritional FTT which supplementation devices they used, why and how well or poorly they assisted in resolving the problem. In each case, ask them to indicate whether/how/why resolution of the problem spelled the end of breastfeeding. (I)

27. Describe ankyloglossia (TR19- 6). Review the frequency of its occurrence and how it is usually managed in your community. (You may need to inquire of dentists, oral surgeons, and/or pediatricians in your area to determine the frequency of occurrence of this problem.) Answer the question: why have many health professionals ceased considering it an issue relative to poor feeding in the past 50 years? (I)

28. Invite three mothers to class to describe their baby's experience with breastfeeding while tongue-tied. (If possible, get one mother whose baby's tongue was clipped soon after birth, one mother whose baby's tongue tie resolved by itself over time, and one for whom problems continued. In each case, ask each mother to describe *her* experience with breastfeeding. (I)

CHAPTER 20

Work Strategies and the Lactation Consultant

This chapter examines the developing profession of lactation consulting and various concerns of the lactation consultant in an institutional setting as well as in private practice in the community. Working as a member of the health care team also is discussed.

KEY CONCEPTS

1. **Assertiveness** - The end result of self-confidence and feeling comforable when presenting oneself and one's views to others. Although this characteristic is considered an asset in men, until recently, this attribute in women has been considered a negative trait by some, particularly those persons who view women's roles as more passive than men's. Nevertheless, being assertive is essential to getting one's views across without also attacking others or being attacked.

2. **Burnout** - A situation in which need/demand for assistance/services exceeds the ability of the helping professional to provide it. In many cases, poor planning contributes to burnout. In other cases, external factors—such as effective advertising, more than expected growth, and the like—contribute to it.

3. **Cash flow** - The amount of money that comes in and goes out of a given office. Incoming cash is considered income; outgoing cash is considered expenses. For a practice to be considered legitimate by the US Internal Revenue Service, income must exceed expenses three years out of five. When it does not, the practice is considered a hobby, not a business, and certain tax benefits of running a business may be lost.

4. **Certification** - the process by which lactation consultants via examination and later by continuing education credits, are objectively determined to have the minimal skills considered essential to offer assistance to breastfeeding mothers and their babies.

5. **Charting** - refers to the recording of key elements in each contact with a client in order to provide complete reports to other health professionals, including referring individuals and—occasionally—third party payors.

6. **Hospital privileges** - The opportunity to see clients in a hospital; usually after acceptance of application for privileges and corroborating support from a professional who already has privileges by the hospital committee(s) governing such activities.

7. **Lactation consulting** - An allied health offering recently recognized in the professional literature, as well as through its own certification program through examination given worldwide. This profession is an outgrowth in many instances of breastfeeding counseling voluntarily offered in the local area, but not always recognized by the professional community.

8. **Legal liability** - The degree to which a professional can be considered responsible for untoward, unanticipated, or other results deriving from her/his actions in assisting a client/patient. In the case of LCs, practice should include the following elements pertaining to legal concerns: permission related to touching, making no guarantees, avoiding the causation of emotional distress, and maintenance of confidentiality. In some cases, LC services are covered by insurance.

9. **Partnership** - One kind of practice in which two or more individuals share responsibilities (all or only some) for a practice. In some cases, only the physical plant is shared. In other cases, all aspects of the practice are shared in more or less equal amounts, usually governed by a contract between the partners. In some cases, the partnership is incorporated.

10. **Politics** - The art of persuading others that what another wants to do is in everyone's best interests. Specific to lactation consulting, playing politics is often an integral part of the experience of proposing, establishing, and maintaining a lactation service.

11. **Rounds** - Providing services or information to patients/clients and/or other health workers. In some cases, such rounds refer to the provision of services, as when an LC does lactation rounds in the hospital, providing assessment and direct care and recommendations to mothers. In other cases, rounds refer to information-sharing as in departmental rounds or grand rounds where one or more persons makes an invited presentation and answers questions from an audience of her/his peers.

READINGS FOR FURTHER REFERENCE

1. Bornmann, P: *Legal Considerations and the Lactation Consultant.* (Unit 3). Lactation Consultant Series. Garden City Park, NY: Avery Publishing Group, 1987.

2. Jensen, D, Wallace, S, Kelsay, P: LATCH: A breastfeeding charting system and documentation tool. *JOGNN* 23:27-32, 1994.

3. Matthew, MK: Mothers' satisfaction with their neonates' breastfeeding behaviors. *JOGNN* 20:49-55, 1991.

4. Matthews, MK: Developing an instrument tossess infant breastfeeding behaviour in the early neonatal period. *Midwifery* 4:154-65, 1988.

5. Mulford, C: The Mother-Baby Assessment (MBA): An "Apgar Score" for breastfeeding. *J Hum Lact* 8:79-82, 1992

6. Riordan, J, Woodley, G, Heaton, K: Testing validity and reliability of an instrument which measures maternal evaluation of breastfeeding. *J Hum Lact* 10:231-35, 1994.

LEARNING ACTIVITIES

1. Review each of the four attributes of an assertive person (see TR 20-1). Provide an example of assertive behavior relevant to the following situations: (I)
   a. Marriage: encounter of husband and wife
   b. Business: encounter between employee and employer
   c. Health care setting
      1) encounter between midwife or nurse and physician
      2) encounter between health worker and client/patient

2. Review "How to Swim with Sharks" (pp.551-52 in the text). Ask the students to relate assertive behavior to each of the elements in the Cousteau piece. (I)

3. Review "Tips for Working with Women Co-Workers in a Work Setting" (TR 20-2). Ask the students to examine each of the seven elements and write a paper discussing one positive and negative aspect of each of the elements. (I)

4. Review the factors that can contribute to burnout. (I)

5. Invite a hospital-based, clinic-based, MD office-based, and private practice LC to participate in a panel discussion of burnout. Ask each person to answer the following questions: (I)
   a. How many hours do you spend in the office?
   b. How many clients per day/per week do you see?
   c. How have you controlled the size of your practice?
   d. In what way(s) have you experienced burnout?
   e. In what way(s) have you attempted to avoid burnout?

6. Explain cash flow; using the following example, show how careful consideration of same is essential to running a successful business. (I)

YEAR 1	Income	Expenses	Cumulative Net Income
Month 1	-0-	$400	(400)**
Month 2	250	—	(150)*
Month 3	100	—	(50)
Month 4	300	100	150
Month 5	350	—	500
Month 6	350	200	650
Month 7	400	50	1000
Month 8	350	—	1350
Month 9	520	—	1870
Month 10	450	—	2320
Month 11	450	200	2470
Month 12	1100	—	3570
TOTAL	4620	950***	3670

* Money amount in () is a loss.
** Money used to obtain supplies; what might these be in an LC business?
***20% of gross income

7. Ask an accountant to explain how the amount of expenses and the amount of gross income must each be assessed to determine the relative "health" of the business in question. (I)

8. Ask a business consultant to discuss those factors that should be considered beforeopening a private practice. (I)

9. Review how lactation consultant certification was developed. (I)

10. Review the seven elements of charting (see TR 20-3). (I)

11. Invite a panel of LCs who have been certified to discuss how they prepared for the certification exam and their impressions of that examination. (I)

12. Have your students review charting options as shown in Appendix B (p. 638), Appendix I (pp.657-64), and Appendix 19-1 (pp.536-40). In each case, the students should note: (S)
    a. information common to all charts; examine two of the three charts to answer this question.
    b. most complete chart; least complete chart, and why students characterize them in this manner
    c. factors considered most helpful in each case
    Also consider in-hospital charting options described by Matthews and Mulford, and Jensen, et al. Then review the Riordan article. Ask your students how these in-hospital charting tools relate to other charts discussed previously.

13. Describe and discuss the two different methods of charting (see TR 20-4) that are discussed in Chapter 20. What method is used in two or three of the hospitals in your community? Are different methods of charting used by level of care provided? What specific charting elements are used to record infant feeding information? (I)

14. Invite a panel of nurses from three or more hospitals in your community to describe how they chart mother-baby care. In each case, each panel member should be asked to explain: (I)
    a. whether they use narrative or problem-oriented charting
    b. whether particular questions pertaining to infant feeding are included; if not, why not? which elements (specific questions and why they are used)
    c. if particular methods of charting are used for infant feeding, what this is, and how this technique was determined to be useful? Is this a technqiue different for bottle-feeding and breastfeeding babies?
    d. Where is infant feeding information placed, and why?
    e. Where is infant feeding information stored after mother and baby are discharged?

15. Ask four (4) LCs to present a panel discussing the pros and cons of hospital privileges; how they obtained them (if they have them); why they do not (if they don't). (I)

16. Ask three hospital-based LCs to describe the degree to which they offer each of the services listed in "Hospital-based Lactation Programs/services" (see Transparency 7). For each, ask them to: (I)
    a. note which services were offered in which order as they program was expanded
    b. identify which services are *not* offered and why
    c. identify which services are a future offering
    d. the role of competition between hospitals in offering certain services

17. Review the history behind lactation consulting and how it developed. (I)

18. Invite an attorney to discuss each of the following issues as it relates to providing LC services (see TR 20-5, 20-6). Invite an LC to be present to provide concrete examples of situations in which these elements might apply: (I)
    a. permission (written and/or oral) before touching the client or her infant
    b. make no promise or guarantee that will not be provided;
    c. avoid causing the mother, the baby, or any other member of the client's family emotional distress;
    d. maintain confidentiality about the mother, baby, and family.

19. Review the advantages and disadvantages of solo practice and partnerships (see TR 20-7, 20-8, 20-9, 20-10). In each case, explain why each element must be considered carefully. (I)

20. Have a panel discussion that includes input from a solo practitioner, a member of a two-person, three-person, or larger practice. Not all may be LCs or LC practices. After each has presented a brief overview of their practice and why they maintain it, ask the class to direct questions to each or all of the panel members. The questions should include: (I)

a. what is the most difficult aspect of running your partnership/business?
b. If you could make the "perfect partner," what characteristics would they have? How many of these characteristics do(es) your current partner(s) have?

22. Explain how different individuals contribute to a political decision to: (I)
    a. propose an LC program
    b. establish a program
    c. maintain a program that is ongoing
    d. expand a program that is ongoing

23. Review the do's and don't's of lactation consulting that pertain to rounds in the hospital. Explain why one should or should not do each of the elements you have highlighted. (I)

24. Ask your students to select a topic for a "grand rounds" presentation pertaining to *any aspect* of lactation consulting on which they wish to focus. They should outline their presentation and then present it for review by their peers. (S)

25. Send your students to a local hospital. Have them interview at least one of the following personnel: (S)
    a. physician (pediatrician or family practitioner)
    b. midwife
    c. nursery nurse*
    d. postpartum nurse*
    e. lactation consultant**

    In each case, the student will ask:
    a) Do you recommend pre-lacteal feeds for breastfeeding babies? bottle-feeding babies? Are they routinely offered in your hospital unit? If so, why? If not, why not?
    b) What problems have you observed with pre-lacteal feeds?
    c) If the hospital's policy has changed from using to not using pre-lacteal feeds, when did this change occur, why was it made, and how do you feel about this change?

* if the hospital uses a mother-baby care arrangement, there may only be one nurse representing these areas
** this person may not work in the hospital in all communities

READINGS FOR FURTHER REFERENCE

Burns, N, Grove, SK: *The Practice of Nursing Research: Conduct, Critique and Utilization, 2nd ed.* Philadelphia: WB Saunders, 1993.

Holcomb, ZC: *Interpreting Basic Statistics.* Los Angeles, CA: Pyrcak Publishers, 1992. Order from: PO Box 39731, Los Angeles, CA 90039.

Roberts, C, Burke, SO: *Nursing Resarch: A Quantitative and Qualitative Approach.* Boston: Jones and Bartlett Publishers, 1989.

Riordan, J: Research for the practicing lactation consultant: where to start? what questions to ask? who can help? *J Hum Lact* 5:78-80, 1989.

LEARNING ACTIVITIES

1. Define data analysis (see TR 21-1). Using the Sample Data Set found on pp. 70-71 following, discuss what kind of analysis is appropriate for understanding... (I)
   a. each variable on its own; ie., to characterize the sample
   b. whether a relationship exists between each independent variable and the dependent variable, breastfeeding duration
   c. whether the relationship(s) found are statistically significant, and whether they are clinically important, regardless of their statistical significance
   d. what generalizations can be made from the sample
   e. what practice recommendations can be made from the findings, if any.

2. Explain why one would use different analyses for different kinds of data. (I)

3. Distinguish between the following data collection techniques, noting the pros and cons of each (Use TR 21-3, 21-4 in your discussion): (I)
   a. document/chart review
   b. laboratory findings
   c. field observation
   d. participant-observation
   e. structured interview
   f. unstructured interview

4. Ask the students to identify four variables about which they wish to collect information. Then ask them to do so using two different techniques of data collection. Their task is to describe the benefits of each technique and their respective limitations for each of the variables whose data they have collected. (S)

5. Describe ethnography and ethnographic research. Provide an example in a culture with which you, the instructor, are familiar. (I)

6. Ask your students to develop an ethnographic study of a subgroup within their culture with which they are familiar. At least four elements in their description should relate to infant feeding. An oral presentation or written paper is the result. (S)

7. Describe grounded theory. Distinguish it from other approaches using the same information. (I)

8. Ask your students to develop a grounded theory based on information they have obtained from 10 or more breastfeeding mothers. Encourage creative thinking. (S)

9. Discuss the development of hypotheses and their relationship to... (I)
   a. theoretical constructs
   b. data to be gathered
   c. data analysis
   d. report of findings

10. Ask your students to write out four different hypotheses pertaining to infant feeding experiences. Ask them to restate their hypotheses in the null form. Then ask them to explain which form they prefer, why, and how each would influence data gathering. (S)

11. Distinguish between two different methodologies by which hypotheses could be tested (refer to TR 21-2). (I)

12. Ask your students to distinguish between quantitative and qualitative methodologies. Using a hypothetical data set, they should then link the data to the methodologies chosen. (S)

13. Describe an operational definition. Link it to data to be collected, illustrating *how* you have selected the particular definition of the variable in question. (I)

14. Discuss the limitations and appropriateness of each of these operational definitions of breastfeeding: (I)
   a. one or more feeds at breast before hospital discharge
   b. a preponderance of feeds at breast within the first three months of life
   c. all feeds at breast each day
   d. feeds at breast with or without solid foods
   e. feeds at breast with or without other fluid feeds
   In each case, how might the findings be affected by each operational definition discussed?

15. What is phenomenology? How does it differ from other theoretical approaches? (I/S) [If you ask the students to write a paper answering these questions, request that they also provide examples comparing phenomenology with other theoretical approaches to illustrate the points they are making.]

16. Ask your students to design a study using the phenomenological approach. What other approach might they select to understand the same life experiences? (S)

17. Distinguish between a population and a sample. (I)

18. Ask your students to develop a technique for (S)
   a. identifying a population; and
   b. selecting a sample from that population. Ask them to do so.

19. Distinguish between a qualitative approach and a quantitative approach. Give examples of each. (I)

20. Ask your students to distinguish between a qualitative and a quantitative approach to the analysis of a data set. Their discussion may form the basis of an oral presentation or a class paper. (S)

21. Define reliability. Use examples that illustrate high reliability and low reliability. (I)

22. Ask the students to use two different techniques to obtain the same information in order to determine the reliability of the data they have gathered. (S)

23. Describe a research problem, linking it to the theoretical construct, the methodology to be used, the data gathering technique, operational definition(s), and planned data analysis. (I)

24. Ask your students to state a research problem. They must then link that statement to: (S)
   a. the theoretical construct
   b. the methodology to be used
   c. the operational definitions to be used
   d. data gathering technique
   e. planned data analysis

25. Explain why review of the literature is important. Examine two publications, one of which does not adequately review the literature and one which does. How is the latter a better presentation of that which has gone before? (I)

26. Ask your students to write a brief review of the literature of a particular problem. Limit their review to ten (10) articles focused on the same issue, all of which are primary references of research endeavors. (S)

27. Review the 1946 Nuremberg trials; how do the rights of human subjects today derive from these trials? (I)

28. Discuss the implications of each of the four rights of human subjects (as described in Key Concept #16). Give an example of each from a research protocol. (I)

29. Ask your students to obtain copies of consent forms from at least two institutions. Compare them. How might they be improved? At local institutions, what kind of protection protocol must all researchers using human subjects endure? If a meeting is held to review such protcols, have your students request an invitation to attend such a meeting as an observer. (NOTE: This may or may not be allowed insofar as such meetings are considered to discuss potentially sensitive and confidential matters; in some cases, the observers may have to leave when votes or recommendations are made.) (S)

30. Define sampling. Give an example using the same original population for each of the following sampling techniques: (I)
   a. network
   b. convenience
   c. solicited
   d. purposive
   e. simple random
   f. systematic
   g. stratified random

   In each case, link the limitations and benefits of each sampling technique to the hypothesis to be tested and the data to be gathered.

31. Ask the students to select three different sampling processes in order to discuss their pros and cons in different situations and for different research questions. An oral or written presentation may result. (S)

32. Define the setting for a research study. How might this be related to the research question to be answered? (I)

33. Ask your students to evaluate a local hospital, a local clinic or physician's office, and a local gathering site for young mothers as an appropriate setting in which to carry out a research study. In each case, they are to examine the pros and cons of each setting and their limitations for conducting a qualitative study, and a quantitative study. (S)

34. Describe validity. How does it relate to reliability? Distinguish between internal and external validity. Give examples of each and how some study designs prevent consideration of validity. (I)

35. Ask your students to distinguish internal and external validity by evaluating published research purporting to provide information related to each. (S)

36. Identify variables and what they are. Distinguish between dependent, independent, extraneous/intervening/confounding variables. (I)

37. Ask your students to evaluate at least five different research articles. In each case, they are to identify dependent, independent, intervening/confounding variables and explain why they have so identified them. (S)

Sample Data Set

Case	Age	Breastfeeding Duration	Marital Status***	Parity**	Work Information*
1	17	3 weeks	Single (S)	1	—
2	17	4 weeks	S	1	—
3	18	5 weeks	M	1	F
4	18	14 weeks	S	2	P
5	19	20 weeks	M	1	P
6	19	19 weeks	M	1	P
7	19	5 weeks	D	2	F
8	20	4 weeks	S	3	—
9	20	14 weeks	M	1	—
10	20	7 weeks	M	1	F
11	21	5 weeks	S	1	P
12	21	3 weeks	M	1	F
13	21	7 weeks	M	2	F
14	22	13 weeks	D	2	F
15	22	20 weeks	M	1	P
16	23	1 week	M	1	—
17	23	17 weeks	M	1	—
18	23	41 weeks	M	2	—
19	24	14 weeks	M	2	P
20	24	15 weeks	S	3	F
21	24	21 weeks	M	1	F
22	25	26 weeks	M	1	F
23	25	28 weeks	M	3	F
24	25	13 weeks	S	3	—
25	25	12 weeks	S	4	P
26	26	27 weeks	M	2	—
27	26	20 weeks	M	2	—
28	26	43 weeks	M	1	F
29	26	5 weeks	M	2	F
30	26	7 weeks	S	1	P
31	26	49 weeks	M	3	P
32	27	52 weeks	M	5	P
33	27	29 weeks	M	2	F
34	27	53 weeks	M	2	P
35	28	3 weeks	S	2	P
36	28	14 weeks	W	3	—
37	29	29 weeks	M	3	—
38	29	64 weeks	D	1	—
39	30	28 weeks	M	2	—
40	30	15 weeks	M	2	—
41	30	10 weeks	S	1	—
42	31	17 weeks	M	2	P
43	31	12 weeks	M	3	P
44	32	57 weeks	M	3	F
45	33	48 weeks	M	3	F
46	34	54 weeks	M	3	F
47	34	5 weeks	M	1	P
48	35	7 weeks	S	1	P
49	35	9 weeks	S	1	F
50	36	47 weeks	M	2	—
51	36	22 weeks	M	3	—
52	36	20 weeks	M	3	—
53	37	59 weeks	D	2	F
54	37	39 weeks	M	1	P

* Work information relates to fulltime employment (F); parttime employment (P). No information can be assumed to mean the woman does not work outside the home.
** Parity 1 means mother has had her first baby; Parity 2 means mother has had her second baby, and so on. (No information is provided for gravida status.)
*** Marital status: Single (S), Married (M), Divorced (D), Widowed (W)

Information Relating to the Sample Data Set

Descriptive Statistics
n=54

	Range	Mode	Median	Mean
Age	17-37	26	26	26.35
Parity	1-5	1	2	1.90
Breastfeeding Duration	1-64 weeks	---	17	22.27

Central Tendency of the Variables
Most women are in their mid- to late-20s
Most women have had their first child (46%)
Most women are married (67%)
Most women work parttime or fulltime (64%); however, the group is nearly equally divided between fulltime and parttime work.

What is the relationship between these variables?

1. Age and marital status: no apparent relationship
2. Age and parity: as age increases, parity increases
3. Age and work status: no apparent relationship
4. Age and breastfeeding duration: women younger than 20 are more likely than older women to breastfeed less than 8 weeks; women 25 years or older are more likely than younger women to breastfeed 6 months or longer
5. Marital status and parity: no apparent relationship
6. Marital status and work status: single women are more likely to work parttime than other women, who are more likely to work fulltime
7. Marital status and breastfeeding duration: single women are more likely to breastfeed less than 5 weeks; married, divorced, and widowed women are more likely to breastfeed 2 months or longer
8. Parity and work status: no apparent relationship
9. Parity and breastfeeding duration: the lower the parity, the shorter the breastfeeding duration

CHAPTER 22

Issues in Human Milk Banking

This chapter examines human milk banking, its history, and how it is currently practiced.

KEY CONCEPTS

1. **Banked human milk** - human milk that is stored for later use. Such milk may derive from one or more women, and may represent different "ages" of milk; it may or may not be pasteurized or treated in some way to retard or prevent the growth of pathogens within the milk.

2. **Cultural issues** - in different cultures, different belief systems govern the acceptability and use of banked human milk. The clinician working with women needs to be aware of such beliefs in order to appropriately recommend the use of banked milk within the context of its cultural acceptability.

3. **Donors of human milk** - one or more persons who provide some portion or all of their milk for use by their own infant or other babies. If other babies are the recipients, usually these infants are unknown to the donors.

4. **Environmental pollutants** - elements that can contaminate human milk which derive from the donor's own environment. Some of these pollutants represent no danger to the infant; in other cases, such environmental contaminants may render her an inappropriate donor, particularly if the recipient infant is ill or otherwise compromised.

5. **Heat treatment** - one means of deactivating certain disease properties that may be found in human milk. For example, pasteurization of human milk kills the HIV organism if it is present, thereby preventing its transfer to the recipient infant.

6. **Marketing banked human milk** - techniques whereby the availability of donor milk is identified for potential recipient infants.

7. **Milk collection** - techniques whereby milk is made available to recipient infants from donor lactating women. Such collection may occur by hand expression or by breast pump.

8. **Milk handling** - techniques employed to preserve the cleanliness of the milk when its transfer is not direct from mother to baby.

9. **Milk screening** - the methods used to determine if the milk has contaminants or disease elements that would render it inappropriate for potential recipient infants.

10. **Milk storage** - techniques used to save the milk for later use. These can include methods for raw fresh, refrigerated, lightly-, or deeply-frozen milk.

11. **Quality assurance procedures** - methods for assuring that donor milk meets certain requirements designed to keep it clean and appropriate for use by recipient infants.

READINGS FOR FURTHER REFERENCE

Arnold, LDW: HIV and breastmilk: what it means for milk banks. *J Hum Lact* 9:47-48, 1993.

Arnold, LDW: Human milk for premature infants: an important health issue. *J Hum Lact* 9:121-23, 1993.

Arnold, LDW, Larson, E: Immunologic benefits of breast milk in relation to human milk banking. *Am J Infect Control* 21:235-42, 1993.

Golden, J: From wet nurse directory to milk bank: the delivery of human milk in Boston, 1909-1927. *Bull Hist Med* 62:589-605, 1988.

Michaelsen, KF, Skafte, L, Badsberg, JH, et al: Variation in micronutrients in human bank milk: influencing factors and implications for human milk banking. *J Pediatr Gastroenterol Nutr* 11:229-39, 1990.

Human Milk Banking Association of North America: *Recommendations for Collection, Storage, and Handling of a Mother's Milk for Her Own Infant in the Hospital Setting.* Order from PO Box 370464, West Hartford, T 06137-0464 USA; (202-232-8809).

Pardou, A, Serruys, E, Mascart-Lemone, F, et al: Human milk banking: influence of storage processes and of bacterial contamination on some milk constituents. *Biol Neonate* 65:302-9, 1994.

Pierce, KY, Tully, MR: Mother's own milk: guidelines for storage and handling. *J Hum Lact* 8:159-60, 1992.

Rayol, MRS, Martinez, FE, Jorge, SM, et al: Feeding premature infants banked human milk homogenized by ultrasonic treatment. *J Pediatr* 123:985-88, 1993.

LEARNING ACTIVITIES

1. Review the history of human milk banking and relate it to the history of breastfeeding patterns worldwide. (I)

2. Ask your students to visit a local human milk bank. If this is not possible, ask them to write one of the milk banks in their country or a neighboring country. Their task is to learn *when* the bank began operation, *how* it is run, *why* it was established, typical donors, typical recipients, and the number of ounces of milk it receives and distributes each year. (S)

3. Review representative cultural beliefs about human milk. Note how these might relate to acceptance or resistance to using banked human milk. (I)

4. Invite 5 women who have donated their milk to a bank to explain why they have chosen to do so. (I)

5. Summarize the variety of environmental pollutants in your area. How are these pollutants handled by the local milk bank? (I)

6. Describe different kinds of heat treatment that a mother might use at home. Invite a milk bank worker to contrast at-home heat treatment with typical milk banking procedures. (I)

7. Ask a milk bank representative to come to class and describe how milk is handled and why it is handled in this manner (refer to TR 22-1). (I)

8. Ask a milk bank representative to come to class and describe how donors and their milk are screened, when such screening occurs, and why such screening is done. (I)

9. Review how milk can be stored and why this may be different at a bank than in a home. (I)

Student Projects That Require Data Gathering

Although activities for students are provided for each chapter in earlier sections of this Resource Guide, the following activities relate specifically to information-gathering that involves questioning breastfeeding mothers or other groups of persons who, as a group, may highlight certain activities and/or insights into the clinical management of the lactation mother and/or her breastfeeding baby.

Undergraduate students should be encouraged to involve a minimum of five individuals (in most cases), but probably no more than 20, keeping in mind both time constraints and degree of sophistication of student understanding of the research process. Graduate students should be expected to increase the minimum number to 25 or more. Much will depend, in this situation, on the statistical analysis planned and the necessary minimum number of cases expected in each cell for each variable to be analyzed.

For both undergraduate and graduate students, the instructor may ask for work additional to that which is suggested in the following project recommendations.

For Chapter 1:

1. Interview 5 breastfeeding mothers to determine what influenced them to breastfeed. For example, interview one woman in each of several of the following settings/circumstances.
    1. a pregnant woman expecting her first baby
    2. a pregnant woman expecting her second or later baby
    3. a mother who had a baby within the past three days (in hospital)
    4. a mother whose baby is now 4 weeks old
    5. a mother whose baby is now 8 weeks old
    6. a mother whose baby is 3 months old
    7. a mother who has returned to work
    8. a mother who gave birth to twins, triplets or quads
    9. a mother whose baby was born prematurely
    10. a mother who bottle-fed an older child and is breastfeeding her most recent baby

2. Interview 5 mothers. Ask them what the mothers think about wet-nursing, if they have known someone who breastfed a baby not born to them, and the circumstances in which the wet-nursing occurred (**NB:** wet-nursing is not the same as induced lactation). Ask each mother if they would or would not consider...
    a. wet-nursing another mother's child;
    b. seeking the services of a wet-nurse for their own baby; and,
    c. under what circumstances they would or not do a) or b) above.
    The outcome of these interviews might serve as a presentation, oral or written, focusing on wet-nursing.

For Chapter 3:

1. Interview 5 families who have recently had a baby. In each case, they should determine:
    a. who visited the mother following her baby's birth (in the hospital/birth center and at home) and were they members of the nuclear, or extended family, or a non-family member?
    b. who is included in the mother's nuclear family? extended family?
    c. what role relationships (if any) are missing in each mother's family?
    d. What strengths/weaknesses of each family can the student identify?
    e. How might those strengths/weaknesses influence
        1) each mother's infant feeding decision-making?
        2) each mother's breastfeeding course?

For Chapter 8:

1. Interview 5 different persons with similar characteristics (e.g., all are teens, all are new mothers, all are African American, etc.). These persons are to be asked the following questions:
   a. how have you decided your baby(ies) will be fed?
   b. when did you make this decision (If you have not decided, when do you think you will decide?)
   c. who influenced your decision?
   d. how were you influenced?
   e. what information would have made you change your mind?
   The results of these interviews will form the basis for a written or oral presentation regarding infant feeding decision-making.

For Chapter 9:

1. Interview 5 breastfeeding women who have had a baby within the last seven days. In each case, they should the student should ask the mother:
   a. Tell me how you knew you had milk.
   b. Did you feel full in your breasts at any time since your baby's birth? If so, when (what day) and how long did it last? If not, why do you suppose you did not feel this fullness?
   c. What were you told to do to reduce the breast fullness you had?
   d. Did anyone call this "engorgement?" Who was that?
   e. What were you told (prenatally, postpartum) about breast fullness and engorgement?
   f. What advice worked well? What advice did not?

2. Ask 5 mothers who have experienced infant breast refusal. (These women could be identified from contact with a lactation clinic, an LC or a mother-to-mother breastfeeding support group in the local community.) In each case, ask the mother to characterize the breast refusal she experienced by answering when it occurred, why she thinks it occurred, and how the refusal was resolved. Specifically, she should be asked...
   a. How did you resolve the refusal? How long did it take before your baby was again breastfeeding? If the baby did not return to the breast, how did she feel about this?
   b. When the baby refused the breast for the first time, what led to the refusal, in the mother's opinion? (Based on the student's gathering of information about the refusing behavior, what is the student's conclusion about precipitating factors for the breast refusal?)
   c. To whom did the mother turn for assistance? What advice that she received was most helpful? unhelpful?
   d. What would the mother tell others in order that they might avoid infant breast refusal?

3. Ask 5 or more women who were identified by others (lactation clinic, private LC, mother-to-mother support group) as having experienced insufficient milk production. In each case, ask:
   a. clinical evidence, if any, prior to weaning that this was the case;
   b. infant behaviors supportive of such a conclusion;
   c. maternal experiences supportive of such a conclusion;
   d. statements by health workers supportive of such a conclusion;
   e. what the mother did to resolve the situation, if anything;
   f. what she would tell other mothers about insufficient milk production.

4. Interview at least 5 women who have given birth within the last two months. Ask them to note:
   a. how many women experienced leaking in the first week? first month? today?
   b. when they experienced leaking (before, during, after breastfeeding)?
   c. how they stopped the leaking from occurring?
   d. whether they wore breast pads? if so, what kinds and with what result?

5. Contact a community group known to support and assist breastfeeding mothers who have given birth to twins, triplets, quadruplets or quintuplets. For at least 5 mothers, inquire about:
   a. the mother's feeding plan before she knew she was having more than one baby
   b. the mother's early breastfeeding experience with her multiples
   c. the mother's later breastfeeding experience with her multiples
   d. differences with multiples compared with breastfeeding a singleton
   e. what problems she encountered and whether and how she resolved them
   f. how the mother would characterize her breastfeeding multiples experience, including whether/how she would
      1) encourage another mother to breastfeed two or more babies
      2) discourage another mother from attempting to breastfeeding two or more babies
      3) avoid the problems she encountered

For Chapter 10:

1. Visit a Level III nursery, and review the charts of 5 different babies being gavage fed. Discuss with the babies' nurses how long their charges have/will be gavage fed, what they are getting by gavage, and the babies' health status, and problems to date.

2. Ask several mothers whose preterm infants have received human milk fortifiers and how they felt about using these items. The results will serve as an oral or written presentation.

3. Inquire how 5 mothers of preterms felt about test-weighing their babies to assess the amount of milk transfer at each feeding. Did they continue to do so after the baby's discharge? If so, how did they feel about continuing such test weighing? The results of these interviews may serve as an oral or written presentation by the student.

For Chapter 11:

1. Ask 5 mothers and at least 5 different breast pump outlet sources (such as a pharmacy, grocery store, breast pump rental depot, lactation consultant, hospital-based lactation clinic, etc) regarding breast pump comfort, use, popularity, and preference. In each case, ask the mothers about the breast pump(s) they use(d) and whether they met the criteria of maternal concern (TR 11-1). If the mothers have used more than one breast pump, ask about the order of breast pump use, why each mother used more than one pump, the relative financial and emotional costs of each, and so on. From those making pumps available, ask about money-back guarantees, pattern of sales/rentals for each pump, and why the particular range of pumps is offered.

2. Interview several mothers who have used breast shells. The following information should be sought:
   a. *who* recommended using breast shells?
   b. *when* was this recommendation made?
   c. *why* was the recommendation made?
   d. *what kind* of breast shell was used?
   e. *what effect* did the breast shells have?
   f. *how long* were the breast shells used?
   g. *what problems*, if any, occurred as a result of breast shell use?
   h. *how* were these problems resolved?
   i. what did the breast shells *cost*? were they *worth* that cost?

3. Ask 5 or more mothers who have used a nipple shield about their experiences. In each case, ask:
   a. *who* recommended use of a nipple shield
   b. *when* it was used
   c. *why* it was used
   d. *how* well/poorly it worked and how long the mother breastfed; do the students infer a relationship between use of a nipple shield and breastfeeding duration?
   e. *problems*, if any, experienced
   f. *recommendations* to others who might use a nipple shield

for Chapter 12:

1. Ask 5 new mothers [their babies are 1-5 weeks old], what they know about jaundice and hyperbilirubinemia and how they gained this information. Write a paper deriving from the mothers' knowledge and understanding of these terms. [**NB**: Do *not* offer explanations or answers pertaining to the topic generally or to a given mother's baby in particular. Instead, encourage the mother to ask for an explanation from a pediatric staff member with whom she has contact.]

2. Interview at least 5 mothers, each of whose baby had late-onset jaundice. Ask the following questions in order to prepare a paper discussing "the influence of late-onset jaundice in the first month of neonatal life:"
   a. *when* was the diagnosis first made?
   b. *who* made it?
   c. *what changes*, if any, in feeding were recommended?
   d. if c above occurred, how did these changes affect
      1) the mother;
      2) her milk supply;
      3) the baby;
      4) the baby's feeding pattern?
   e. *how long* was the baby considered to have late-onset jaundice?
   f. What would the mother want other mothers of babies similarly diagnosed to know about:
      1) the condition;
      2) how it was managed;
      3) its effect on feeding;
      4) its effect on maternal nurturing?

3. Ask 10 staff members at one or more hospitals about water supplementation and the role it plays in routine care plans for breastfed and artificially-fed infants. Their interviews could form the basis of oral presentation, term paper, or both.

for Chapter 13:

1. Interview 5 women with one of the following health problems and identify the similarities and differences in their treatment and their breastfeeding course:
   a. asthma
   b. diabetes (gestational)
   c. diabetes (IDDM)
   d. hyperthyroidism
   e. hypothyroidism
   f. multiple sclerosis
   g. postpartum depression
   h. seizure disorder

for Chapter 14:

1. Conduct a survey of 5-20 physicians and 5-20 nurses in the area regarding their knowledge about the incidence, symptoms and suggested treatment of women with mastitis during lactation.

for Chapter 15:

1. Interview several mothers in different employment settings about their decision(s) to use (or not) a breast pump and what concerns/factors went into their decision-making. The results of these interviews could form the basis of an oral presentation, a term paper, or both.

2. Interview 15 women with children under two years of age (5 mothers with one child, 5 mothers with two children, and 5 mothers with three or more children). The purpose is to determine how maternity leave available to them affected their decision regarding return to work. .

3. Interview 5 mothers in front of the class regarding their breastfeeding pattern at different times with their babies. Ask the students to characterize the mothers' experiences. Was there a "pattern" to the baby's feeds? If so, how might it be described? If there was no pattern, how might that affect the at-home mother? the employed mother?

4. Ask how 5 different mothers coped with fatigue during the first week, the first month, the first year of parenthood. How was breastfeeding related to their fatigue? How was maternal employment related? What did they do to cope? How much sleep did they usually get? At times other than night, how much sleep/rest time did they get?

for Chapter 16:

1. Ask at least 5 women who have breastfed at least 12 months about the duration of their lactation-related amenorrhea. The resulting paper will discuss the variables relating to the women's experiences, including:
   a. frequency of suckling at 1st month, 3rd month, 6th month, etc.;
   b. duration of suckling episodes at 1st month, 3rd month, 6th month, etc.;
   c. timing of cessation of night feeds (sleeping at least 6 hours);
   d. timing of introduction of solid foods.
2. Survey at least 5 women. The topic is "How did supplemental feeding influence your baby's breastfeeding pattern?" Questions should include:
   a. when did baby receive first supplemental feed?
   b. was it added to or a substitute for breastfeeding?
   c. what was that first supplemental feed?
   d. how often did these occur?
   e. when did you begin menstrual cycling?
   f. how often, after supplemental feeding was begun, did the baby breastfeed?
   g. age of baby at the time of total weaning from the breast?

for Chapter 17:

1. Survey 5-20 mothers of infants 6-12 months old. Inquire of thier baby's reaction to strangers who come into the house; who meet them on the street. How has this reaction changed over time?

for Chapter 19:

1. Interview 5 women, each of whose baby has been identified by an LC as having a disorganized suck. Ask:
   a. how baby sucked when first put to breast?
   b. when baby's suck was first identified as disorganized?
   c. whether the mother had sore nipples?
   d. how the mother felt when she first learned what the problem was?
   e. how long did it take before the baby's suck was organized?
   f. how was the baby encouraged to use an organized suck?

2. Chart 5 exclusively breastfed and 5 exclusively artificially-fed infants through the first six months of life. What patterns emerge from such charting? Is there a difference in growth patterns by type of artificial milk used to feed the babies who are not breastfed?

3. Ask 5 women, each of whose baby was found to be gaining poorly. In each case, ask about the following factors:
   a. management issues, including limited duration of each feeding bout, inadequate number of feedings/day, inappropriate positioning;
   b. infant factors, including disorganized suckling, neurologic dysfunction, ankyloglossia; and,
   c. maternal factors, including hypothyroidism, maternal drug use (licit and/or illicit), insufficient glandular tissue, poor let-down reflex due to fatigue, caffeine, smoking.

for Chapter 20:

1. Interview at least 3 LCs in the local community (at least one of whom is *not* a nurse or midwife, nor hospital-based) to explain how they became LCs and where they think the field is moving.

2. Interview 2 different LCs who are employed in a hospital-based lactation service. In addition to other questions, ask the following: (S)
   a. who was the "prime mover" in getting the program underway?
   b. who among chairmen, supervisors, administrators are your strongest allies? source of greatest antagonism? behind-the-scenes nitpickers? day-to-day allies?
   c. how have you overcome negatives encountered along the way?
   d. if your service is now expanded, when did you do this, why did you do this, and how did you decide to expand in this way?

for Chapter 21:

1. Collect information on up to five variables from 20 women who have breastfed within the past year.
   a. State the question supporting collection of the information to be asked.
   b. Justify the decision to collect the data in he specific manner chosen.
   c. State how the data will be analyzed.

2. Select an operational definition of breastfeeding and thenobtain information from 10 or more mothers within the framework of that definition. Report how useful/difficult it was to obtain the data within the framework of their operational definition.

for Chapter 22:

1. Interview 5 bottle-feeding women, 5 breastfeeding women, and 5 grocery store managers about their willingness to buy, or sell—respectively—banked human milk if it was made available on store shelves, as is artificial baby milk.

2. Interview at least 2 women in each of three different cultures. Each is to be interviewed to determine how beliefs about human milk in their culture might be related to their views about banked human milk. An oral or written presentation could derive from these interviews.

3. Ask at least 5 breastfeeding mothers whose babies are younger than 2 months whether they would be willing to collect milk if a local milk bank was established. In each case, the students should learn under what circumstances, the mothers would be:
   a. willing to donate their milk
   b. unwilling to donate their milk

AUDIO-VISUAL RESOURCES

Audio-visual materials about breastfeeding and related issues are being produced at a rapid rate. Because there are so many, videos are listed alphabetically; recommendations for use with particular chapters are offered, but need not limit their use with other material. Slide series and other resources are keyed to specific chapters, but may also be used to highlight elements in other chapters as well.

<u>VIDEOS</u>

Baby Friendly Hospital Initiative, 1993 (slide series: Brazil (#C92); Kenya (#C76); Thailand (C95) - $20 each set of 20 slides; Philippines (C92) - $25 (80 slides)
UNICEF, UNICEF House
Division of Information — Photo Unit
3 UN Plaza, H-9F
New York, NY 10017 (212-326-7265)
[for Chapter 1, Chapter 2]

Baby Talk: The Video Guide for New Parents, 1992
VHS, 60 minutes, $28.50
Polymorph Films
118 South Street
Boston, MA 02111
[Chapter 8, Chapter 9]

Breastfeeding: Better Beginnings
11 minutes, VHS, $250
Lifecycle Productions
PO Box 183
Newton, MA 02165
[Chapter 9]

Breastfeeding...For All the Right Reasons, 1989
12 minutes, VHS, $6
Indiana Breastfeeding Promotion Project
1330 West Michigan Avenue
Indianapolis, IN 46206-1964
[Chapter 2, Chapter 8]

Breastfeeding and Accessories, VHS
24-64 min. each; set of 6 videos
1987, Vol. 1 ($29.95); Vols. 2-6 ($6 each)
Medela, Inc.
PO Box 660
McHenry, IL 60050
[Chapter 11]
Capitol Heights, MD
[Chapter 8]

Breastfeeding: A Global Priority, 1990, VHS, $40 (for all four films); individual copies may be free in certain circumstances
UNICEF, UNICEF House
Division of Information — Radio, TV and Film Unit
3 UN Plaza
New York, NY 10017
[for Chapter 1, Chapter 2, Chapter 5]

Breastfeeding...An Individual Experience, 1993,
VHS, 20 minutes, Aus$50
Materntiy\Murwillumbah District Hospital
PO Box 821
Murwillumbah, NSW 2484, Australia
[Chapter 2, Chapter 9]

Breastfeeding: Protecting a Natural Resource, 1990, VHS, 15 minutes (free on request)
Institute for International Studies in Natural Family Planning
Georgetown University Department of Obstetrics and Gynecology
Pasquerilla Healthcare Center, 3rd floor
3800 Reservoir Road NW
Washington, DC 20007
[Chapter 1, Chapter 2]

Breastfeeding: A Special Relationship, 1991
24 minutes, VHS and 3/4" U-matic ($179 for institutions; $79 for individuals)
2201 Woodnell Drive
Raleigh, NC 27603-5240
[Chapter 9]

Breastfeeding Techniques That Work!, 1986-89, VHS, $40 each
Volume 1: First Attachment, 14 min.
Volume 2: First Attachment in Bed, 15 min.
Volume 3: First Attachment after Cesarean, 26 min.
Volume 4: Burping the Baby, 18 min.
Volume 5: Successful Working Mothers, 56 min.
Volume 6: Hand Expression, 18 minutes
Volume 7: Supplemental Nursing System, 23 min.
Geddes Productions
10546 McVine Avenue
Sunland CA 91040
818-951-2809
[Chapter 9]

Breastfeeding, Try It!, 1991, VHS, 4 minutes
Ashland County Ohio WIC
801 Orange Street
Ashland, OH 44805
[Chapter 2, Chapter 8]

Breastfeeding: You Can Make a Difference, 1990
VHS, $7 + shipping
Texas Department of Health
Metropost
501 North 1H-35
Austin, TX 78702

Breastfeeding Your Baby, 1989
VHS, 58 minutes, $11.95 (includes manual)
Medela, Inc.
PO Box 660
McHenry, IL 60050
[Chapter 8]

Breastfeeding Your Preterm Baby, 1989
8-16 minutes, Parts 1,2, and 3; $90 each
Entire set with handout and poster: $200
Health Services Center for Education Resources
Distribution Center SB-56
University of Washington
Seattle, WA 98195
[Chapter 10]

A Challenge to Care: Strategies to Help Chemically Dependent Women and Their Children,
VHS, 38 minutes
Vida Health Communications, 6 Bigelow Sreet
Cambridge, MA 02139
[Chapter 13]

Delivery Self Attachment (Depicts newborn's ability to crawl up to the breast and attach uassisted)
VHS or Beta, 6 minutes, $14.95. English only
Geddes Productions
10546 McVine Avenue
Sunland CA 91040
818-951-2809
[Chapter 9, Chapter 17]

Early Parent-Infant Relationships, 1991, VHS, 25 minutes, $60, purchase only
Developed by Seattle/King County Health Department
March of Dimes
Materials and Supply Division
1275 Mamaroneck Ave
White Plains, New York NY 10605
[Chapter 3]

Healthier Baby by Breastfeeding, 1991
20 minutes, VHS, $19.95
Television Innovation Company
8349 Arrowridge Road, Suite N
Charlotte, NC 28273
[Chapter 9]

Hello Parents!, Adapting to Parenthood, VHS, **length?** $295 Purchase
VIDA Health Communication
6 Bigelow Street
Cambridge, MA 02139
(617) 864-4334
[Chapter 3, Chapter 8]

Helping a Mother to Breastfeed - No Finer Investment. VHS, color - 20 min., $45.
Healthcare Production, Ltds, 1990
Breastfeeding Support Consultants,
164 School House Road, Pottstown, PA 19464
215-326-9343
[Chapter 9, Chapter 13]

Infants and Their Families
(Depicts behavioral differences among infants & how differences influence parenting)
VHS, 23 minutes, Purchase only.
March of Dimes, Materials and Supply Division
1275 Mamaroneck Ave, White Plains, NY, 10605
[Chapter 17]

L'Art de L'Allaitment, 1993 (French only) VHS, 3-part, 55 minutes total, Can$30 + shipping and handling
Part 1: La Nature Fait Blan Les Choses - 16 1/2 min.
Part 2: Un Art Qui SÁpprend - 20 1/4 min.
Part 3: Au Jour Le Jour - 18 min.
Video Femmes
Lígue La Leche
C.P. 874, Saint Laurent, Québec, Canada H4I 4W3
(514) 747-9127 or (514) 747-6667
[Chapter 2, Chapter 8, Chapter 9]

Loving Way/ La Manera Carinosa, 1984, VHS
8 min. ($100) Englis/Spanish
Mattson Multi-Media
11926 Radium Street
San Antonio, TX 18216; (512) 349-3674
[Chapter 2, Chapter 9]

Outside My Mom, 1984, VHS (also available as a slide set)
15 min., $20
March of Dimes
1275 Mamaroneck Avenue
White Plains, NY 10605

Subtle Aspects of Breastfeeding, 1989, VHS
18 min., $30
Breastfeeding Productions
110 Prefontaine Avenue
Seattle, WA 98104

Successful Pumping with the Nurture III, 1991, VHS
9 min., $11.50
Bailey Medical Supplies
1820 Donna Avenue
Los Osos, CA 93402

Supplement Nursing System (Feeding Tube Device)
VHS or Beta
23 min., $39.95 (English and Spanish)
Geddes Productions
10546 McVine Avenue
Sunland, CA 91040

Yes, You Can Breastfeed/Si, Puede dar Pecho, 1990, VHS
13 1/2 min., $7.50 + $3 shipping
Metropost
Attention: ECHO
906 East 5th
Austin, TX 78702

Your Baby: A Video Guide to Care and Understanding, 1989
75 minutes, VHS and Beta, $29.95 + $3.45 (shipping)
Sydney Place Communications
PO Box 6866
Beverly Hills, CA 90212-6866
[Chapter 17]

OTHER AUDIO-VISUAL RESOURCES

Chapter 1
Slides
Baby Friendly Initiative, 1992 (13 color slides or 13 transparencies) $15 each set
Lactation Consultants, Inc.
11320 Shady Glen Road
Oklahoma City, OK 73162

Chapter 2
Slides
UNICEF House
3 United Nation Plaza
New York, NY 10017
Yvonne Simmonds, Photo Librarian 212-326-7265

Chapter 4
Slides
Breastfeeding: An Illustrated Introduction, $60 (includes anatomy and physiology of lactation)
Childbirth Graphics
Division of WRS Group, Inc.
PO Box 21207
Waco, TX 65792
800-299-3366 x287. Fax 817-751-0221

Breast Model
Cost $30.
Childbirth Graphics
Division of WRS Group, Inc.
PO Box 21207
Waco, TX 6579
800-299-3366 x287. Fax 817-751-0221

Chart Set
Full-color charts. (Includes anatomy and physiology of lactation) $60
English and Spanish available
Childbirth Graphics
Division of WRS Group, Inc.
PO Box 21207
Waco, TX 65792
800-299-3366 x287. Fax 817-751-0221

Chapter 9

Audio cassette

Breastfeeding Your Baby 1988, 30 min/side; $20
Medela, Inc.
PO Box 660
McHenry, IL 60050

Softly, Softly—Relaxing to Breastfeed, 1992, 60 minutes, (Aus)$15.95+$15 overseas freight
Merrily Merrily Enterprises
PO Box 231
Nunawading, VIC Australia 3131
(02) 873-1422

The Womanly Art of Breastfeeding, An Audio Guide, 1987, 3 hours on 2 cassettes, $16
LLLI
PO Box 4079
Schaumburg, IL 60168-4079 USA;
(708) 519-7730; (708) 519-0035 fax

Slides

Early Feeding, 20 slides ($20)
Assessing the Infant at Breast, 20 slides ($20)
Frequency of Breastfeeding and Milk Supply, 20 slides ($20)
Sore Nipples, 35 slides ($35)
Engorgement, 18 slides ($18)
1992, All 113 slides ($100)
Lactation Consultant Services
11320 Shady Glen Road
Oklahoma City, OK 73162

Alternative Feeding Methods ($20)
Correct and Incorrect Latch-On ($25)
Premature Infants at Breast ($30)
Positions: Cradle hold, Australian hold, twins ($20)
Definitions of Charting Terms ($15)
Georgetown University Hospital
National Capitol Lactation Center
3800 Reservoir Road NW
Washington, DC 20007 USA
(202) 784-MILK

Chapter 14

Slides

A collection of Breasts (Two slide sets available). $69 for one set, $124 for both.
Geddes Productions
10546 McVine Ave.
Sunland CA 91040
818-951-2809

Audiotape

Barnett. Breast Surgery and Breastfeeding. 1990 Conference and Annual Meeting. Lactation Consultant Association, July, Scottsdale, Arizona
Audiotape # A495, $10.
First Tape, Inc.
770 N. LaSalle St., Suite 301
Chicago, IL 60610

Panel discussion: Product Liability and Lactation Consultants in the US. July 1993 ILCA Conference.
Audiotape #D774, $10. Order: First Tape, Inc., 770N. La Salle Street, Suite 301, Chicago, IL 60610;
312- 642-7793; 312-642-9624 fax

Birth and growth of a hospital breastfeeding program. 1993 ILCA Conference. Audiotape #D776, $10. Order: First Tape, Inc., 770N. La Salle Street, Suite 301, Chicago, IL 60610;
312- 642-7793; 312-642-9624 fax

Care Plans and Protocols

National Capitol Lactation Center. Protocols available for 19 of the most common problems and 12 nursing care plans. $25
Georgetown University Medical Center
3800 Reservoir Road NW
Washington, DC 20007; (202) 784-MILK

EDUCATIONAL COURSE OFFERINGS

The following listing is complete as of the date of publication of this Resource Guide. It includes only those courses that offer more than 15 Contact Hours. Numerous other programs are also available; some offer fewer contact hours; others were unknown to the authors at the time of publication. Persons seeking such education pertaining to lactation and breastfeeding knowledge are encouraged to contact the programs directly for detailed information about what is included in each course, the cost, course length, and other relevant issues. Inclusion on this list in no way implies endorsement by the authors as to the quality of the program offerings.

BREASTFEEDING SUPPORT CONSULTANTS
Director: Judith Lauwers, MA, IBCLC
164 Schoolhouse Road
Pottstown, PA 19464 USA
(215) 822-1281 or (215) 326-9343
Two course offerings:
1 - Breastfeeding Counselor Correspondence Course, 77 contact hours
2 - Lactation Consultant Correspondence Course, 219 contact hours

DOUGLAS COLLEGE PERINATAL PROGRAM
Director: Kathleen Lindstrom
PO Box 2503
New Westminster, BC V3L 5B2 Canada
(604) 527-5478
One course offering:
Breastfeeding Counsellor Certificate Program 12-week course, 30 contact hours; also includes 38 observational hours

EVERGREEN HOSPITAL MEDICAL CENTER
Director: Molly Pessl, BSN, IBCLC
12040 NE 128th Street
Kirkland, WA 98034 USA
(206) 899-2680
Two course offerings:
1 - Basic Course for Lactation Specialists, 42 contact hours
2 - Clinical Preceptorships, contact hours not granted

FLORIDA HEALTHY MOTHERS, HEALTHY BABIES COALITION
Director: Carol Brady, Executive Director
15 Southeast First Avenue, Suite A
Gainesville, FL 32601 USA
(904) 392-5667
One course offering:
Model Hospital Policies and Protocols to Support Breastfeeding Mothers (Training Program for Hospital Staff), approximately 18 contact hours

GEORGETOWN UNIVERSITY HOSPITAL
Director: Vergie Hughes, BSN, IBCLC
3800 Reservoir Road NW
Washington, DC 20007 USA
(202) 784-6455
Two course offerings:
1 - Lactation Consultant Training Program, 36 contact hours
2 - Clinical Traineeship, 100 contact hours

LACTATION INSTITUTE/PACIFIC OAKS COLLEGE
Director: Chele Marmet, MA, IBCLC
16161 Ventura Blvd.
Encino, CA 91436 USA
(818) 995-1913
Three course offerings:
1 - Lactation Educator Program, 30 contact hours
2 - Lactation Consultant Program, 135 contact hours
3 - BA or MA degree in Human Development with specialty in Human Lactation, 165 contact hours in the degree program

LACT-ED, INC.
Course Coordinator: Alison Hazelbaker, MA, IBCLC
5095 Olentangy River Road
Columbus, OH 43235 USA
(614) 459-6313
One course offering:
Lactation Consultant Exam Preparation Course, 43 contact hours

LACTATION PROGRAM
Director: Marianne Neifert, MD
Presbyterian/St. Luke's Medical Center
501 E. 19th Street
Denver, CO 80203 USA
(303) 869-1881
One course offering:
Lactation Program Clinical Preceptorships, 80 contact hourse

MCV/VCU PERINATAL OUTREACH
Director: Cheryl Nunnally, BSN, RN
Medical College of Virginia
PO Box 34
Richmond, VA 23298-0034 USA
(804) 786-5949
Two course offerings:
1 - Symposium for Lactation Training, Course 1
2 - Symposium for Lactation Training, Course 2

UCLA EXTENSION SERVICE
Department of Health Sciences
Directors: Ida Bird, RN, MS and Sandra Steffes, RN
10995 LeConte Avenue, Room 614
Los Angeles, CA 90024 USA
(310) 825-9187
Two course offerings:
1 - Lactation Educator Training Program 44 contact hours
2 - Lactation Consultant Training Program 88 contact hours

WELLSTART
Director: Audrey Naylor, MD, DrPH
4062 First Avenue
San Diego, CA 92103 USA
(619) 295-5192
One course offering (US only):
Lactation Management Education Program, 96 contact hours

WESLEY LONG COMMUNITY HOSPITAL
Director: Maria Sienkeiwicz-Brown, RN, IBCLC
501 N. Elam Avenue
Greensboro, NC 27402 USA
(919) 854-6380
One course offering:
Breastfeeding Educator Program, 23 contact hours

TRANSPARENCY/OVERHEAD MASTERS
Table of Contents

The transparency masters in this listing are designed for use by the instructor to aid in leading discussions, and in elaborating upon material in *Breastfeeding and Human Lactation*. Where the transparencies relate to student assignments or projects, they may also be used to illustrate key points of those assignments or projects. They may be freely copied for such use.

TR 19 - 3 Pattern of Growth Over Time (Duration of Feeds)
TR 19 - 4 Parenting Quotation
TR 19 - 5 Problems Relating to Slow Infant Weight Gain

TR 20 - 1 The Assertive Worker
TR 20 - 2 Tips for Working with Women Co-Workers
TR 20 - 3 Charts and Records
TR 20 - 4 Methods of Charting
TR 20 - 5 Legal Considerations when Providing LC Services
TR 20 - 6 Avoid Legal Liability
TR 20 - 7 Solo Practice - Advantages
TR 20 - 8 Solo Practice - Disadvantages
TR 20 - 9 Partnerships - Advantages
TR 20 - 10 Partnerships - Disadvantages

TR 21 - 1 Problems Appropriate for Scientific Inquiry
TR 21 - 2 Criteria for an Experimental Study
TR 21 - 3 How Researchers Facilitate Clinical Practice
TR 21 - 4 How Clinicians Facilitate Research

TR 22 - 1 Different Human Milk Preparations

Breastfeeding Slogans

- Affordable Health Care Begins With... Breastfeeding
- Be a Producer, Not a Consumer: Breastfeed
- Breastfeeding is Every Baby's Birthright
- Breastfeeding: Lifestyle for Health
- Grow a Brighter Baby: Breastfeed

Breastfeeding Slogans

- If the Baby Could Choose, the Choice Would be Breastmilk!
- Immunize Your Baby Every Day: Breastfeed
- Keep in Touch: Breastfeed
- Mother's Milk: The Highest Quality Product at the Lowest Possible Price
- Babies Deserve the Breast

Promotion, Support, and Protection of Breastfeeding

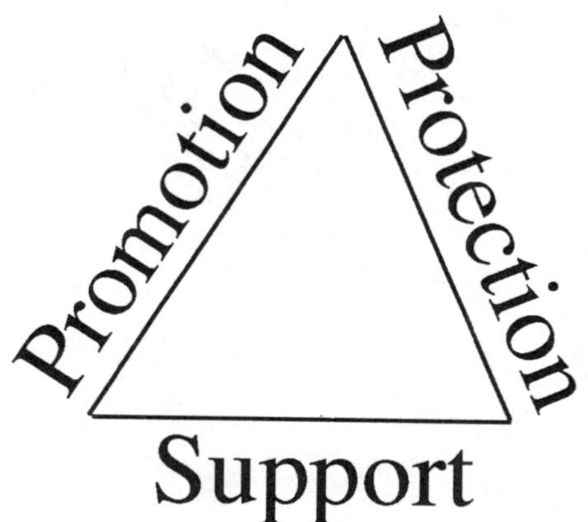

Mother and Infant Needs Intersect

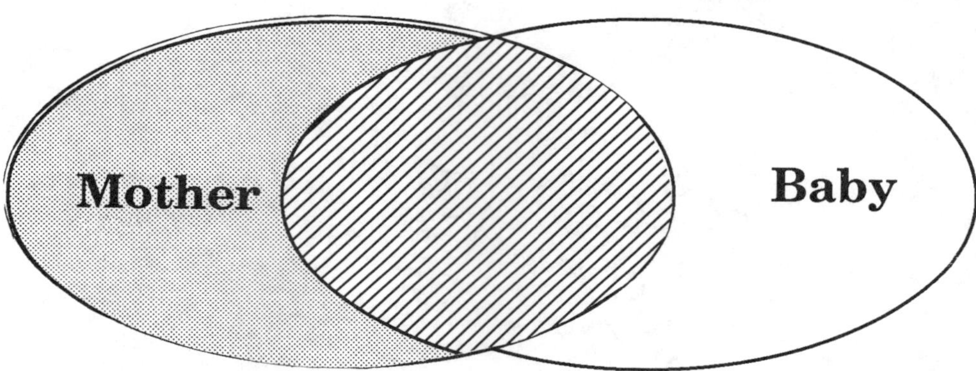

Although each person is an individual, their interaction requires recognition/acceptance of the many ways in which each acts with the other. Most of their early postbirth activity involves both individuals.

WHO Code of Marketing of Breast-Milk Substitutes

- No advertising to the public.
- No free samples to mothers.
- No promotion of products to health-care facilities.
- No company mothercraft nurses to advise mothers.
- No gifts or personal samples to health workers.
- No words or pictures idealizing artificial feeding, including pictures of infants, on the products.

WHO Code of Marketing of Breast-milk Substitutes

- Information to health workers should be scientific and factual.
- All information on artificial feeding, including labels, should explain the benefits of breastfeeding and the costs and hazards associated with artificial feeding.
- Unsuitable products, such as condensed milk, should not be promoted to babies.
- All products should be of a high quality and take into account the climatic and storage conditions of the country where they are used.

Guide for Assessing Culture

- General
- Communication
- Family
- Health Practices
- Religion
- Social Political Systems
- Infant Care Practices
- Infant Feeding Practices

Types of Weaning

- Gradual Weaning
- Deliberate Weaning
- Abrupt Weaning

Family Relationships

Couple Relationship

Wife ______________________________ Husband

Family Relationships

One-Child Family

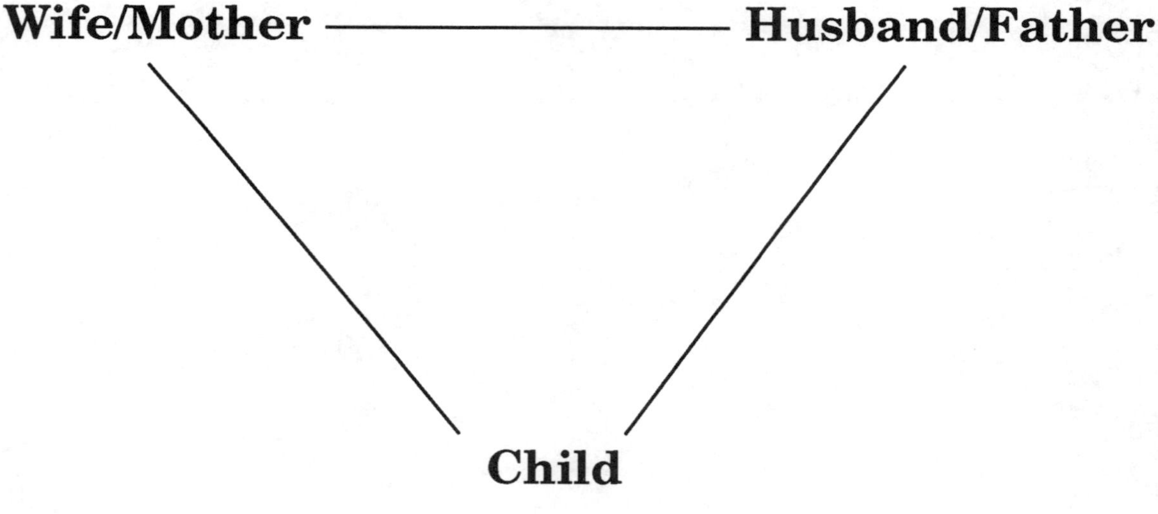

Wife/Mother — Husband/Father

Child

Family Relationships

Two-Child Family

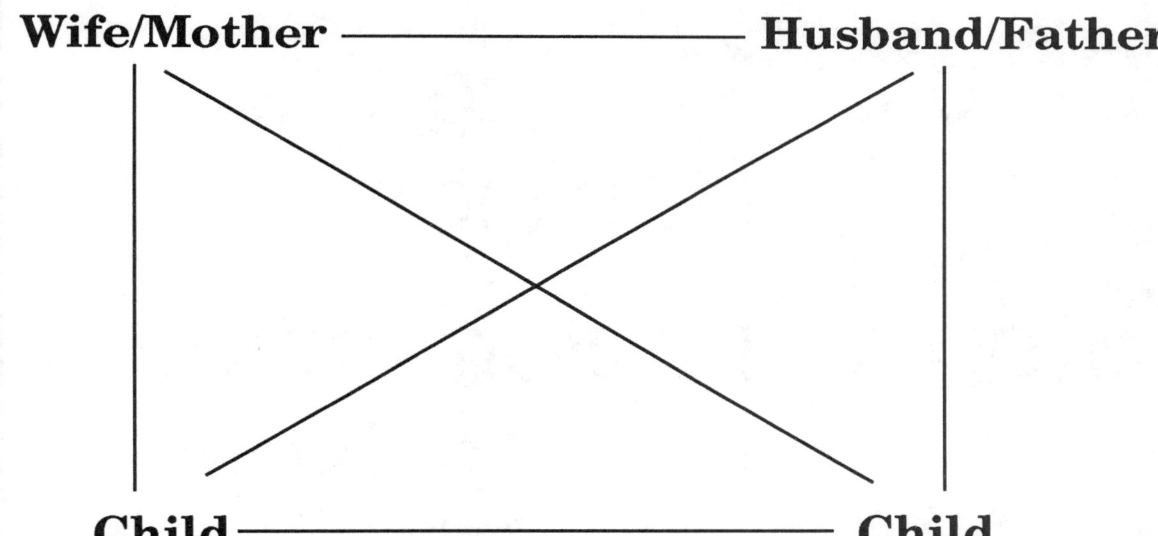

Innovation Decision-Making Process

Step 1: Knowledge

Step 2: Persuasion

Step 3: Making the Decision

Step 4: Implementing the Decision

Step 5: Confirming the Decision

Breast Structure

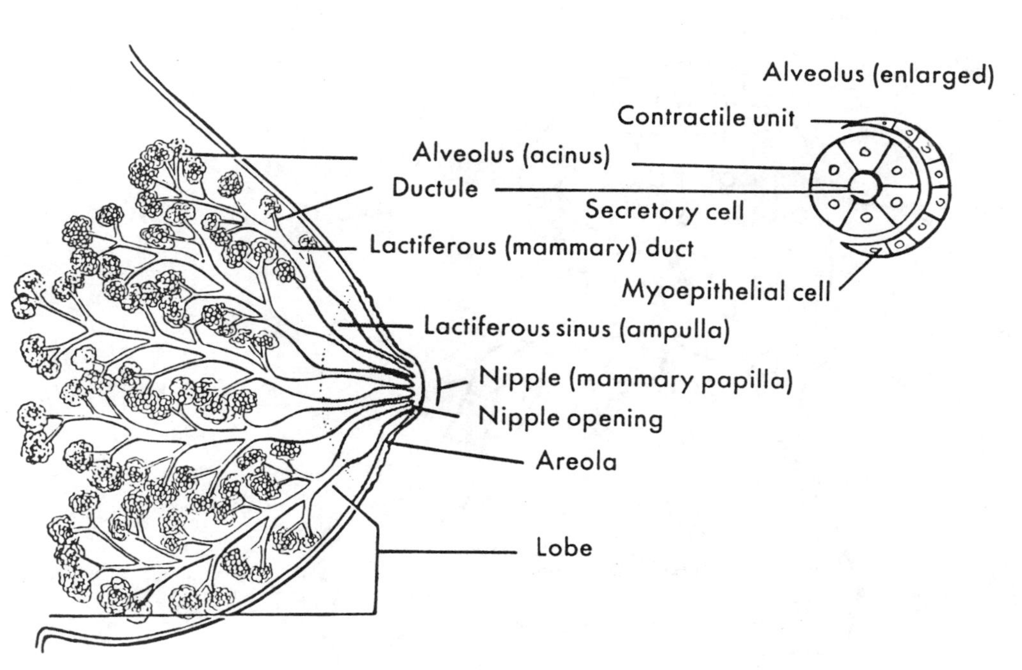

Schematic diagram of breast.

Release and Effect of Prolactin

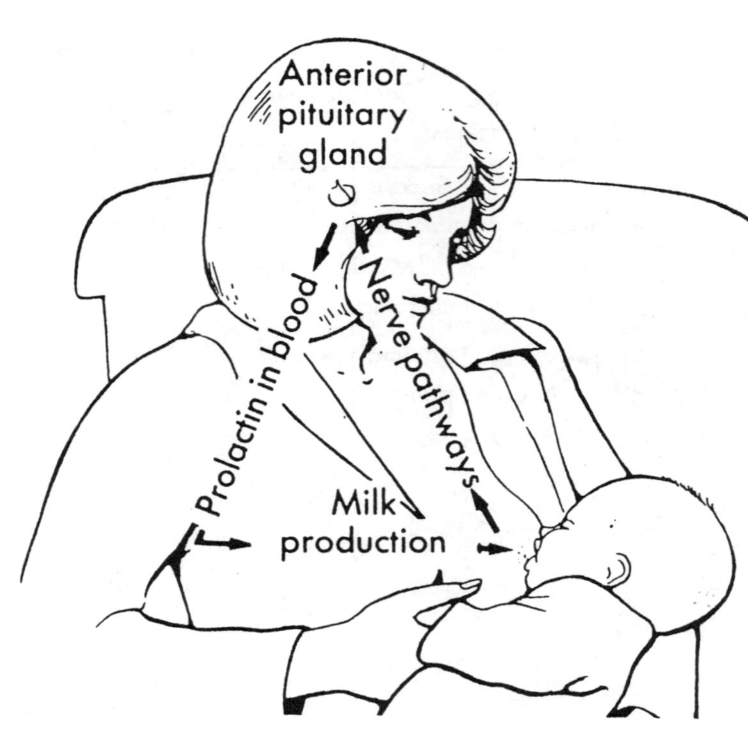

Release and Effect of Oxytocin

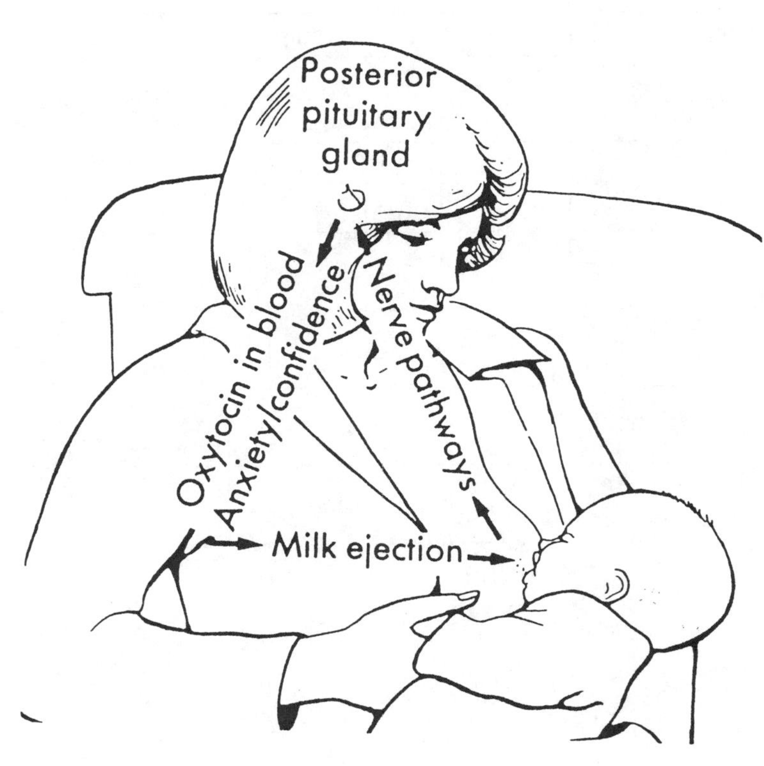

Hormone Levels During Pregnancy and Lactation

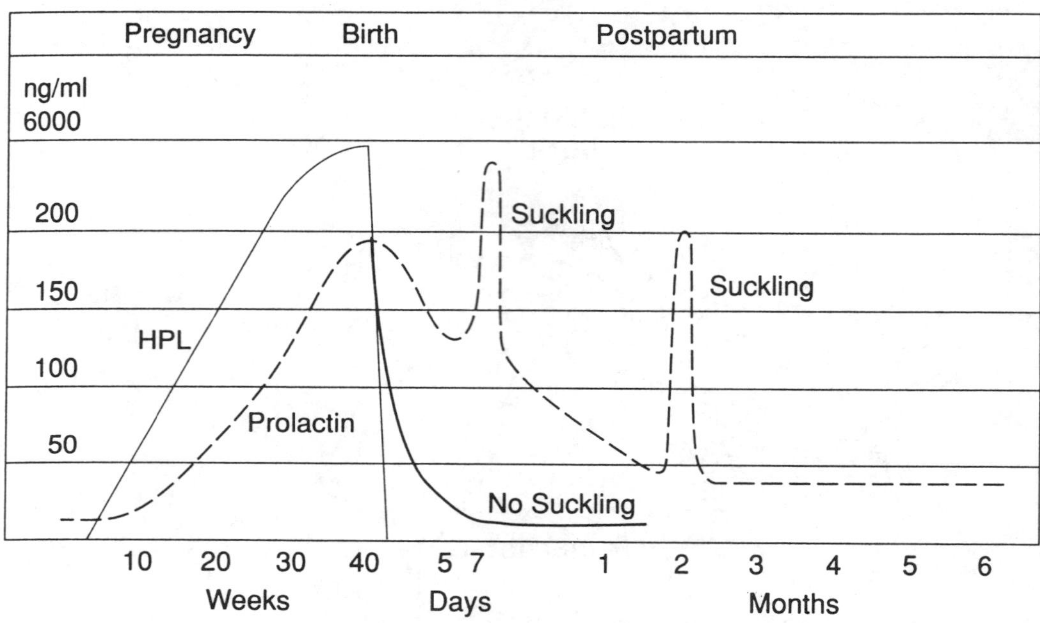

Fluctuation of HPL and Prolactin Serum Levels during Pregnancy and Lactation

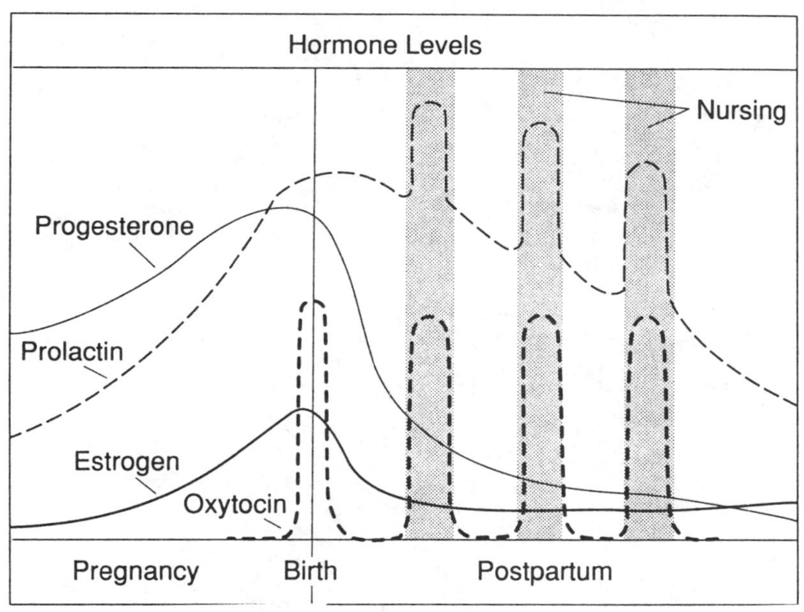

Nipple Retraction

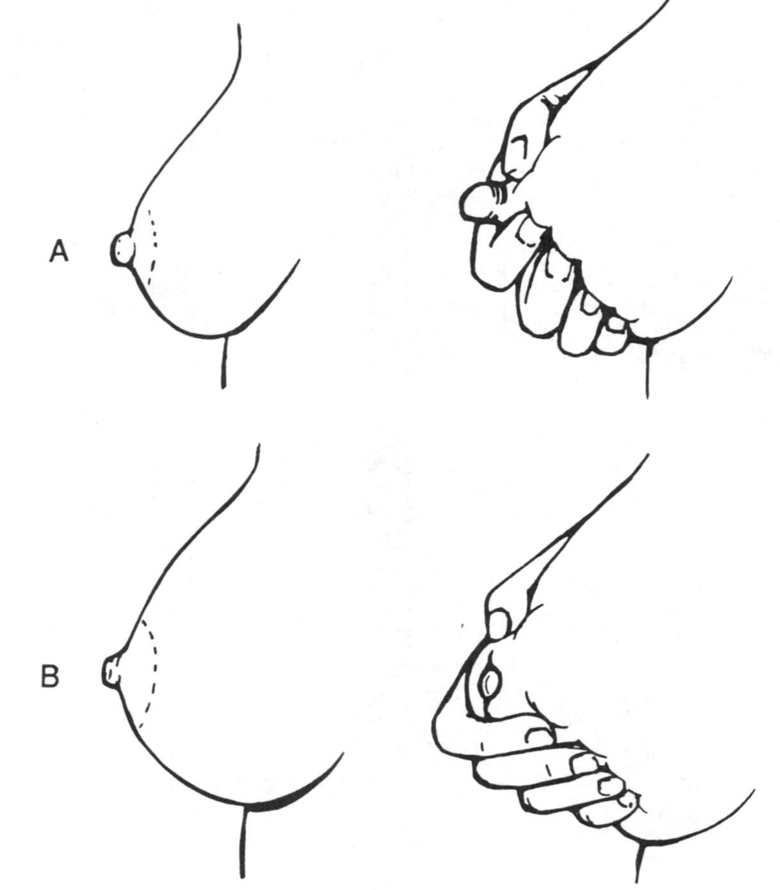

A. Normal Nipple Protraction
B. Moderate Retraction

Nipple Inversion

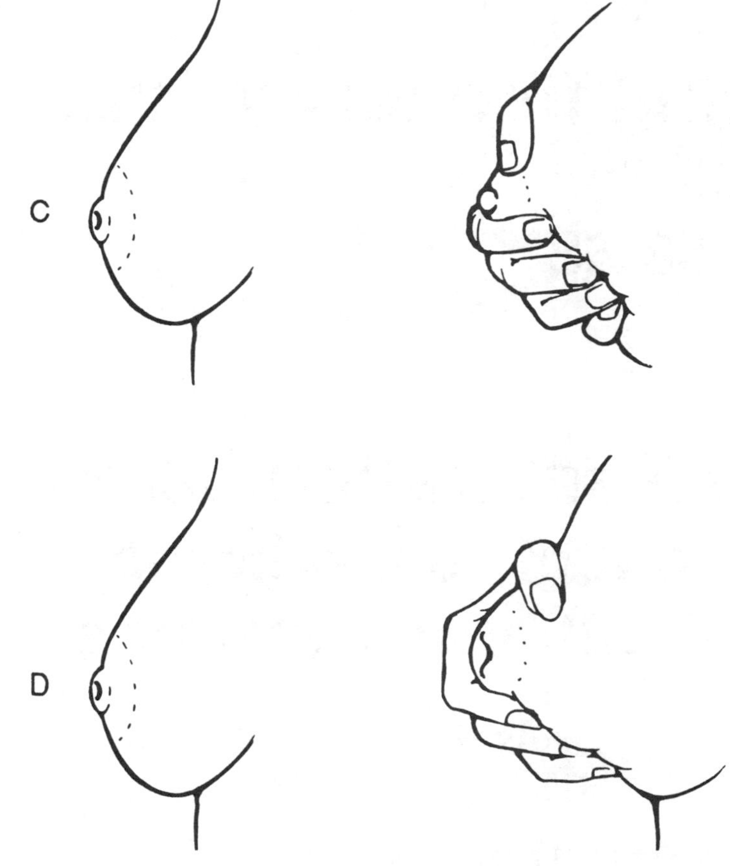

C. Nipple appears to be inverted, but everts with pinch test
D. True inversion

Comparing Breastfeeding and Bottle-feeding

Suckling frequency/min:
- **Brf: 80-88**
- **Bo-f: 58-63**

Oxygen saturation below 90%
- **Brf: 2 out of 10 newborns**
- **Bo-f: 5 out of 10 newborns**

Bradycardia
- **Brf: 0 out of 10 newborns**
- **Bo-f: 2 out of 10 newborns**

Comparing Breastfeeding and Bottle-feeding

Infant's lips

- Brf: flanged outward to make seal
- Bo-f: close together

Mandibular action

- Brf: extensive
- Bo-f: minimal

Tongue action

- Brf: grooved around nipple
- Bo-f: thrust upward and forward

Midsagittal Section of Cranial and Oral Anatomy of Infant Swallow

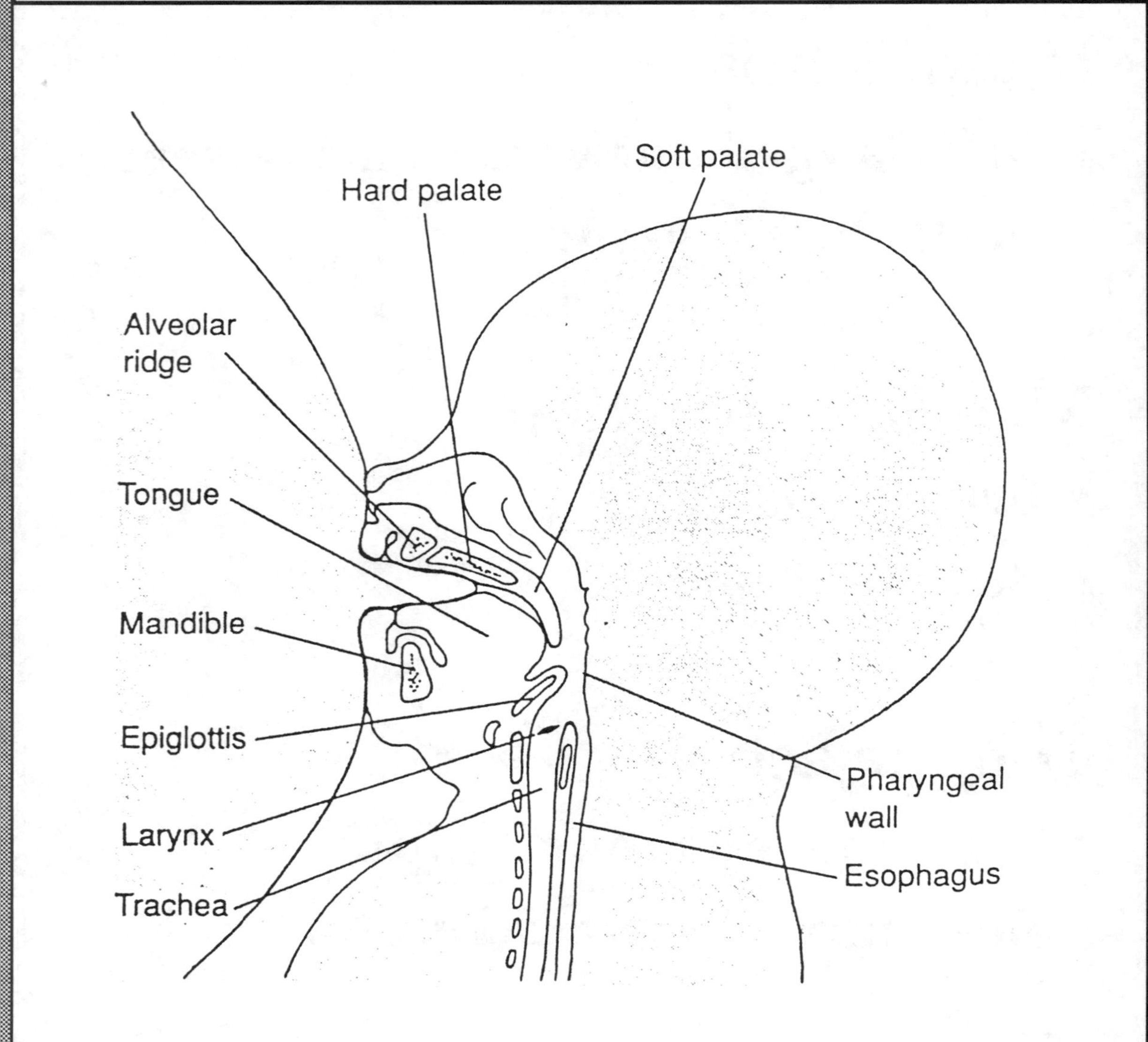

Midsagittal Section of Cranial and Oral Anatomy of Adult Swallow

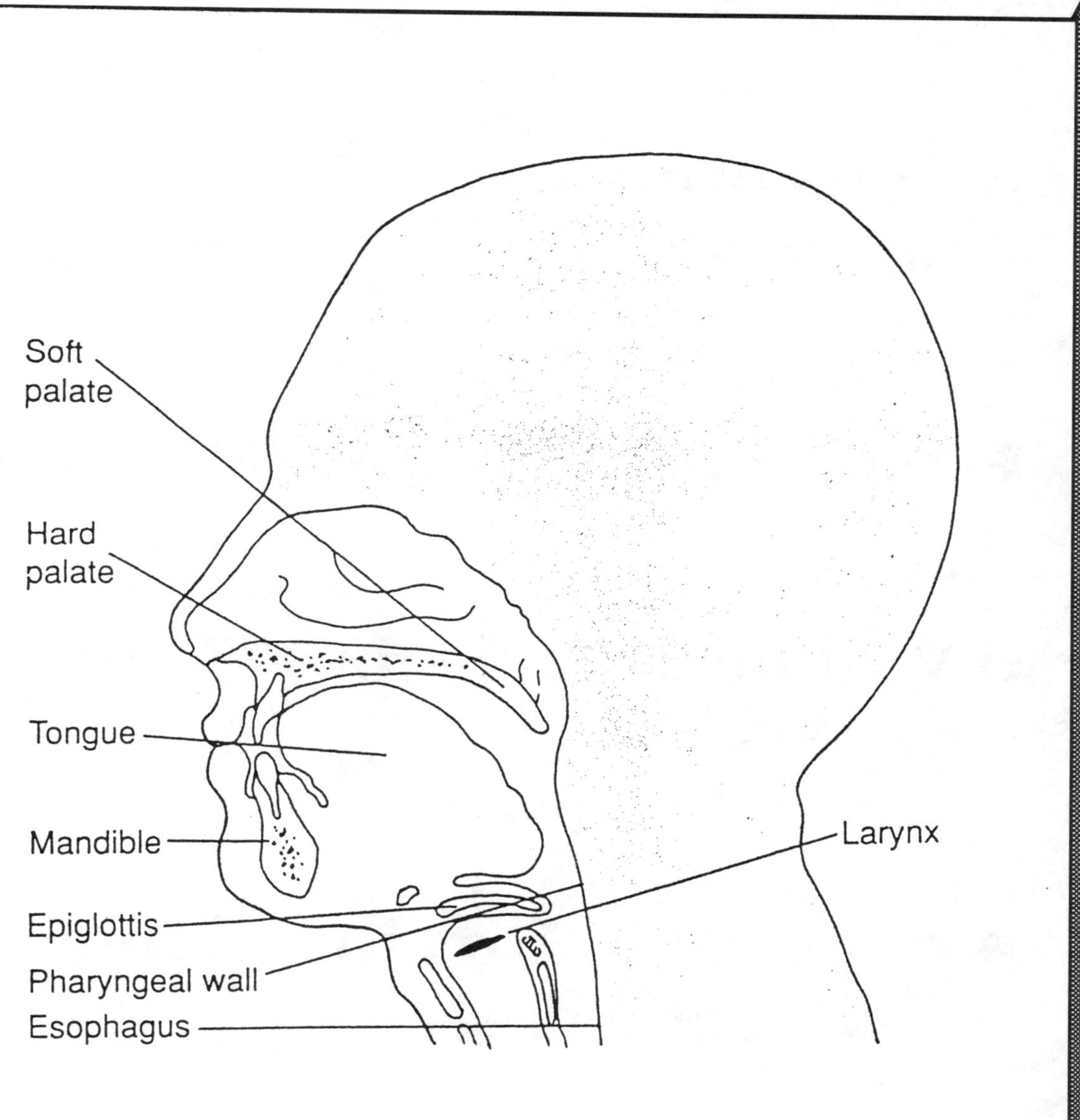

Breastmilk Volume

- Colostrum intake first 24 hours: 37ml (range: 7-123 ml)
- Volume by day 5: ~500ml/day
- Volume by 3-5 mo: ~750ml/day
- Wide variability in volume in different women

Growth in the Breastfed Infant

- First 4 weeks: 10g/kg/day (5-7 oz/ wk
- Weight gain is slightly higher than artificially-fed infant for first 3-4 months
- Weight gain slightly slower than artificially-fed infant after 4 months
- After two years of age, weights are comparable in breastfed and artificially-fed infant

Anti-infectious Factors in Human Milk

- Bifidus factor
- Complement C3, C4
- Inferon
- Lactoferrin
- Lactoperoxidase
- Lymphocytes
- Lysozymes
- Macrophages
- Oligosaccharides
- Prostaglandins
- Secretory IgA

Factors that Affect Drug Transmission

- Molecular Weight
- Plasma vs. Lipid Binding
- Ionized vs. Non-Ionized Molecule
- Acid vs. Alkaline Base
- Half-life
- Milk/Plasma Ratio

Virus Infections

Virus	Breastfeeding Recommended?
Cytomegalovirus	Yes
Herpes Simplex	Yes, if no breast lesions
Rubella	Yes
HIV	Not in developed countries
Chickenpox	Yes

The Change Process

- Assess current situation
- Identify the problem
- Recruit interdisciplinary task force members
- Select target objective(s)
- Select criteria to measure outcome(s)

The Change Process

- Assess likely personnel, system change
- Select action course
- Develop flow chart of action sequence and time frame
- Assign actions
- Create peer support group

The Change Process

- Support, coordinate, supervise to ensure assignment completion
- Evaluate process, outcome
- Revise plan
- Accept change
- Evaluate effects of change

Principles of Breastfeeding Education Programs

- Content, timing coincides with parent readiness to learn
- Information is prioritized, in easily understood and mastered segments
- Anticipatory guidance is practical, realistic
- Printed, visual materials reinforce individual assessment, teaching
- Breastfeeding support resources are identified

Communication Techniques

- Accept
- Give recognition
- Offer self
- Give broad openings
- Make observations
- Encourage descriptions, perceptions
- Encourage comparison
- Reflect feelings
- Rocus and relate
- Give information
- Seek clarification
- Summarize, encourage evaluation

Differences Between Breast Fullness and Engorgement

Characteristics	Fullness	Engorgement
Onset of Symptoms	2-4 days	2-10 days
Site	Bilateral	Bilateral
Swelling	Generalized	Generalized
Heat	Occasional	Generalized
Pain	None - Rare	Generalized
Palpation of Breast	Soft - Firm	Hard
Breast Tenderness	None	Generalized
Body Temperature	<38•C	>38.4•C
Maternal Symptoms	Feels Well	Discomfort, Breast Tightness

Insufficient Milk: Infant Signs

- Baby is restless or irritable during or between feedings
- ...acts "hungry all the time," sucks fists or blanket, moves head rapidly from side to side at breast
- ...comes off the nipple frequently
- ...cries or is fussy constantly, is difficult to console, is fussy right after a feeding
- ...takes baby milk from a bottle right after a feeding
- ...falls asleep at the breast
- ...feeds less than 15-20 minutes on either or both breasts

Insufficient Milk: Maternal Signs

- Mother's breasts feel soft before each feeding
- ...did not enlarge, become tender during pregnancy
- ...did not become full or engorged postpartum

- Mother does not feel milk ejection reflex
- ...cannot express much milk (or less than previously)
- ...has been told that frequent feedings indicate a decreased supply
- ...was told not to put baby to breast if she has cracked nipples
- ...reports previous breast surgery

Assessing Infant Suckling

- What do the baby's cheeks look like?
- Where is the baby's tongue?
- What do you hear when the baby is suckling?
- How tight is the baby's seal on the breast?

Breastfeeding Management for Preterm Infants

- Expression and Collection of Mother's Milk
- Gavage Feeding of Expressed Mothers' Milk
- In-Hospital Breastfeeding Management
- Post-discharge Consultation

Step-by-Step Process for Breastfeeding Premature Infants

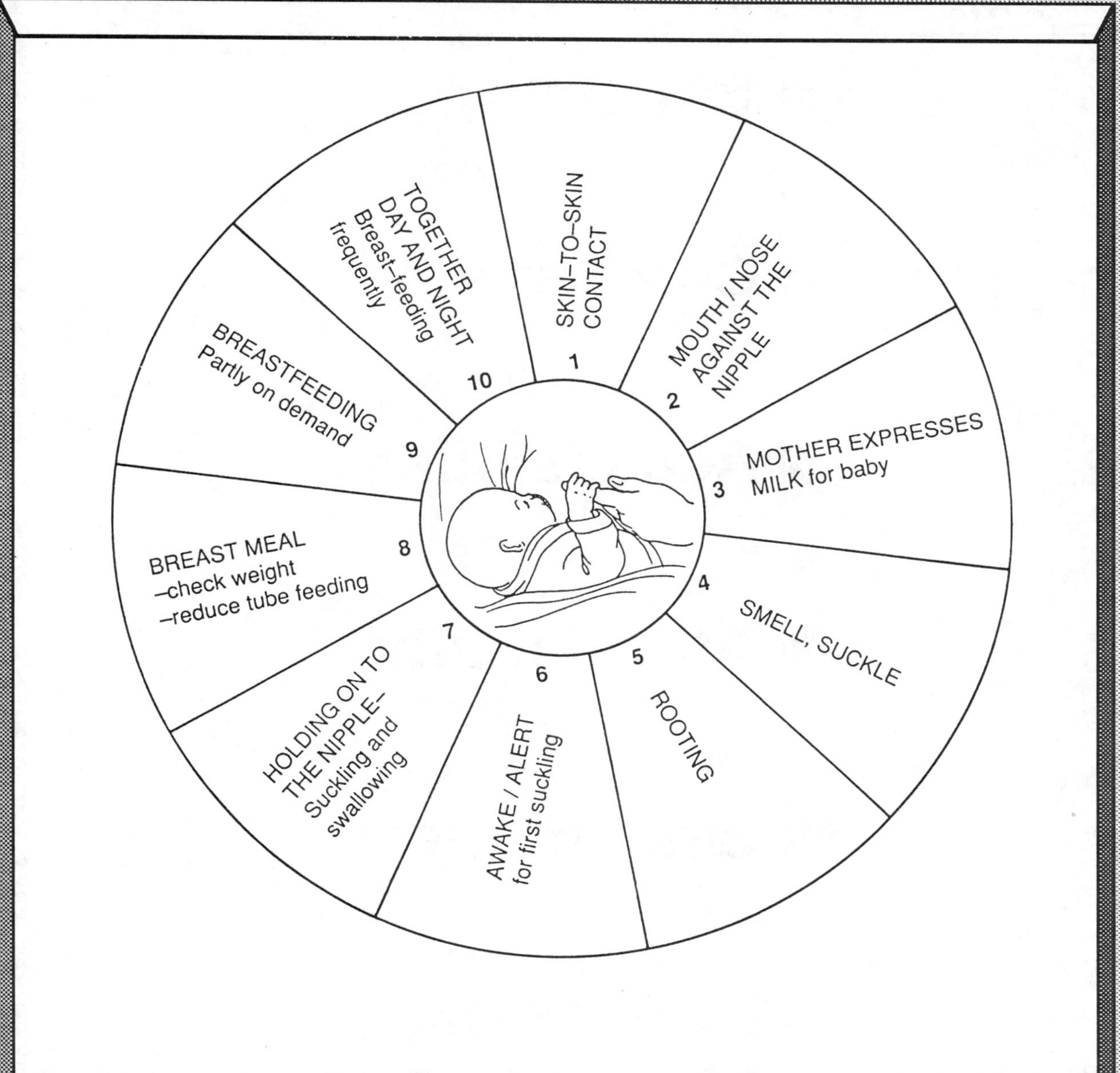

Concerns of Mothers When Using a Breast Pump

- Efficiency
- Comfort
- Accessibility
- Affordability
- Easy to Clean
- Easy to Use

Recommendations for Using a Breast Pump

- Read the Instructions for Using and Cleaning the Pump
- Wash Your Hands Before Using the Pump
- Pump Frequently
- Pump 10-15 minutes (electric); 10-20 minutes (manual)

Technique for Using a Breast Pump

- Elicit milk ejection reflex first
- Use only as much suction as is needed
- Massage breast in quadrants during pumping
- Allow sufficient time to avoid anxiety
- Use inserts to obtain best fit to breast
- Avoid long periods of uninterrupted vacuum
- Stop pumping when milk flow is minimum/nil

Concerns of Professionals About Breast Pump Use

- Most Appropriate Pump for the Situation
- Safe Collection of Milk
- Techniques to Express Milk with Low Bacteria Counts
- Appropriate Pumping Instructions
- Emotional Toll (on Mother) of Expressing Milk

Feeding Tube Systems: Uses for Infant Problems

- Hyperactivity or Hypoactivity
- Down syndrome
- Prematurity
- Cardiac Problems
- Cleft lip/palate
- Perinatal Asphyxia
- Nipple Confusion/Preference
- Neurological Impairment
- Low, Slow, or No Weight Gain, or Weight Loss from Ineffective Suckling
- Lethargy

Feeding Tube Systems: Uses for Maternal Problems

- Adoptive/Foster Nursing
- Relactation
- Breast Surgery
- Primary Breast Insufficiency
- Severe Nipple Trauma
- Contraindicated Medications
- Maternal Illness, Surgery, Hospitalization
- Flat/Inverted Nipples and Infant Inability to Latch

Nipple Shield Use

- To latch onto...
  - Flat nipples
  - Everted nipples when baby does not actively draw nipple into mouth
  - Human nipples following previous use of artificial nipples
  - Engorged breast
- To ease feeding when baby has weak, disorganized, or dysfunctional suck
- To protect sore or damaged (cracked) nipples
- To prevent sore nipples (unproven claim by manufacturers)

Characteristics of Early-Onset Jaundice

- Affects nearly all newborns
- Becomes apparent after 24 hours
- Usually peaks on days 3 or 4
- Declines steadily through the first week
- May be more obvious when feeding is limited in frequency, duration, and when non-milk supplements/complements are used
- Is self-limiting in healthy, fullterm infants
- Requires no intervention

Characteristics of Late-Onset Jaundice

- Affects very few breastfed newborns
- Excludes all pathologic causes
- Infant is thriving, healthy, growing
- Becomes evident in the second week of life
- Peaks around 10 days or later
- Bilirubin level drops rapidly if other milk is given with, or as a substitute for, mother's milk
- Often occurs in all siblings
- Requires no intervention

Assessing Feeding and Jaundice

- How often is the infant being put to breast?
- Is the baby suckling when put to breast?
- Has the baby begun stooling; if so,how frequently is it occurring?
- Is the baby receiving complementary, supplementary feeds?
- Is the mother encouraged to nurse the baby at night?

Health Benefits to Mother from Breastfeeding

- Lower insulin needs if diabetic; better control of blood sugar levels
- Lower risk of developing ovarian cancer
- Lower risk of developing pre-menopausal breast cancer
- Rapid postpartum uterine involution
- Rapid return to pre-pregnant weight

Induced Lactation/ Relactation Considerations

- Primary reason for doing so?
- Time since last breastfeeding/pumping?
- Mother's definition of "success"?
- Family support/opposition?
- Acceptability of use of a device to feed the baby?
- Reproductive history?
- Importance of milk production?

Postpartum Depression

- History of inability to cope with stress
- Lack of social support and/or partner support
- Constant fatigue and lack of sleep
- Mood swings, weepiness, anxiety

Types of Postpartum Depression

- Postpartum "blues" - Transient tearfulness, usually on third day postpartum (70-80% of women)
- Postpartum depression - Mild to moderate clinical depression (20% of women)
- Postpartum psychosis - Irrational, self-accusatory, insomnia, hallucinations (rare)

Medications for Postpartum Depression

Drug	Use/Safety Level
Alprazolam	With caution
Diazepam	With caution
Amitriptyline	Apparently safe
Desipramine	Relatively safe
Imipramine	Relatively safe
Nortriptyline	Apparently safe
Phenelzine	Contraindicated
Tranylcypromine	With caution
Chlorpromazine	Relatively safe
Mesoridazine	Relatively safe
Perphenazine	Apparently safe
Thoradazine	Relatively safe

Medications for Postpartum Depression

Drug (Trade Name)	Use/Safety Level
Xanax	With caution
Valium	With caution
Elavil	Apparently safe
Norpramin	Relatively safe
Trofanil	Relatively safe
Pamelor	Apparently safe
Nardil	Contraindicated
Parnate	With caution
Thorazine	Relatively safe
Serentil	Relatively safe
Trilafon	Apparently safe
Mellaril	Relatively safe

Reducing Radiation Exposure

- Verify that the diagnostic test is necessary
- Reduce dose to minimum
- Use radiopharmaceutical with the lowest known milk concentration and shortest half-life

Classification of Mastitis

- Milk stasis
- Noninfectious inflammation
- Infectious mastitis

Breast Surgery

- Augmentation
  - Infra-submammary
  - Periareolar technique
  - Transareolar
  - Axillary
- Mastopexy
- Reduction
  - Pedicle
  - Free-nipple

Breast Lift/ Mastopexy

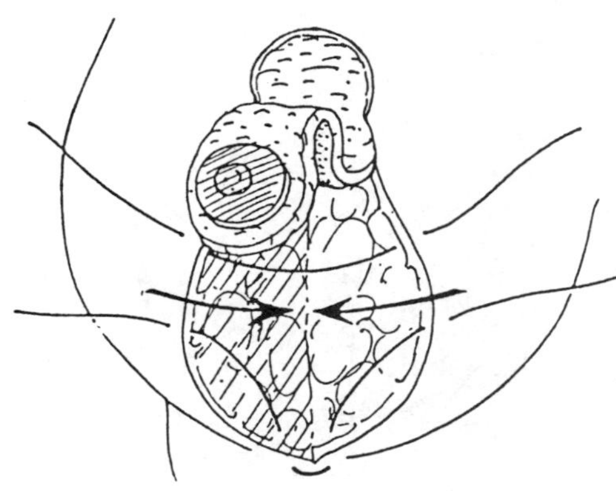

A. Wedge of breast tissue removed, areola pulled up, gap closed

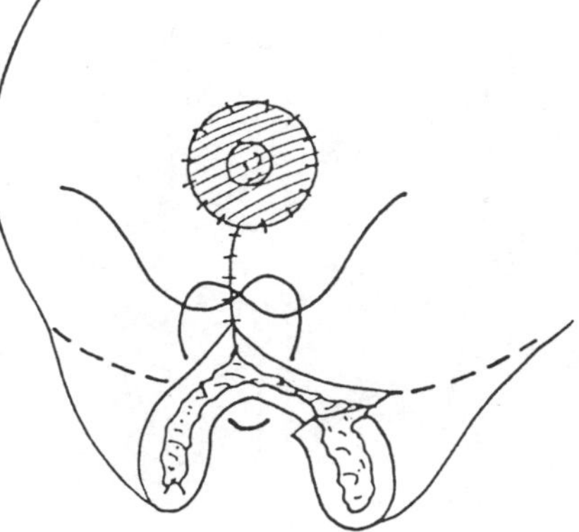

B. Excess tissue removed, skin closed with stitches

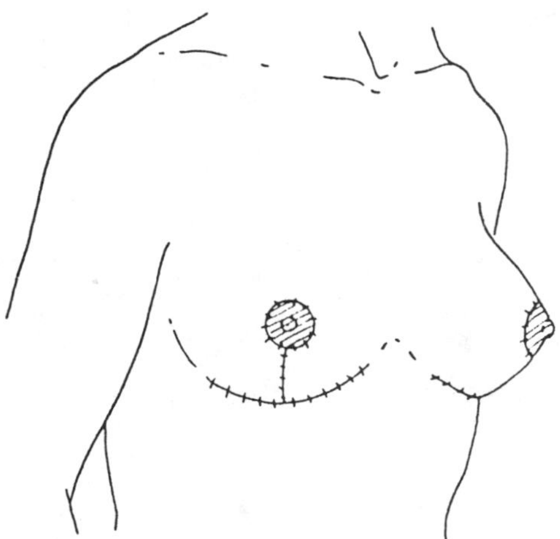

C. Post–operative appearance

Breast Reduction

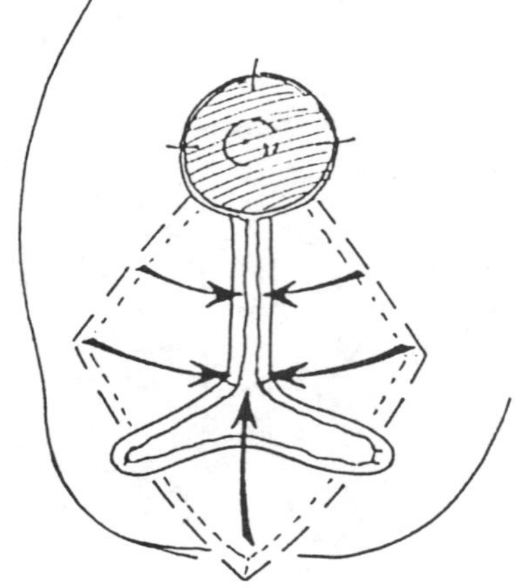

A. Skin edges pulled together

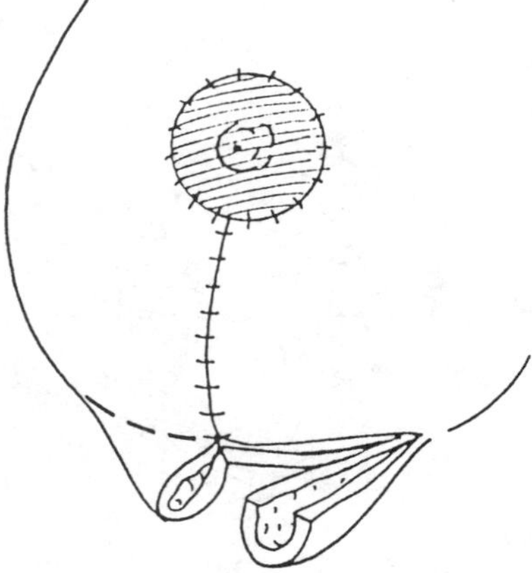

B. Excess tissue removed

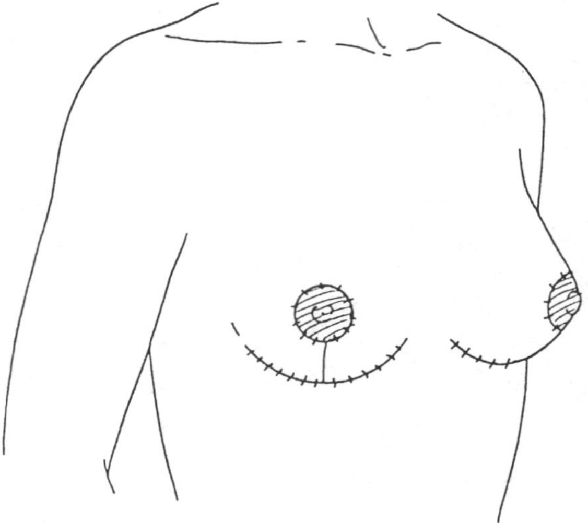

C. Post–operative appearance

Treating a Plugged Duct

- Breastfeed often
- Begin feed on affected breast
- Apply moist heat or soak breast
- Massage affected breast
- Avoid constricting clothing

Checklist for Sore Nipples

- √ **Allow nipples to air after feeding**
- √ **Position baby on arola not nipple**
- √ **Hold infant "chest to chest"**
- √ **Assess for *candida*/thrush**
- √ **Begin feed on least sore side**
- √ **Rotate infant's position at breast**
- √ **Assess for sensitivity to nipple ointment, creams, soaps**

Checklist for Breast Pain

- √ Assess pain intensity and length
- √ Assess for *candida*
- √ Assess for breast constriction, straps
- √ Warm, wet compresses; shower
- √ Express enough milk to soften breast
- √ Gently massage breast prior to feeding

Concerns of Employed Mothers

- fluctuating milk supply
- breast leaking/engorgement
- emotional lability
- need to express milk at work
- baby's need for frequent feeding
- baby's changing feeding pattern

Pumping Questions of Employed Mothers

- Is the pump...
  - easy to clean, use?
  - comfortable to use?
  - effective in obtaining milk quickly?
- What is the initial, continuing cost of use?
- Are instructions for use easy to understand?
- Are replacement parts available?
- Are single/double option kits available?
- Other mothers' reports?

Feeding Options for the Employed Mother

- Breastfeeding
- Cup-feeding
- Spoon-feeding
- Bottle-feeding
- More than one of the above

Barriers to the Employed Breastfeeding Mother

- Lack of child care at/near workplace
- Conditions of work setting
- Employer policies
- Societal attitudes
- Maternal lack of information
- Health professionals' lack of understanding/ knowledge

Sources of Social Support

- A person who cares about the mother and what she wants to do
- A role model
- A knowledgeable advisor
- A person who values breastfeeding
- A person on whose shoulder the mother can lean

Day Care Options

- In-home care
- Family day care
  - sponsored/supervised home
  - regulated
  - unregulated
- Center day care

Decisions of the Employed Breastfeeding Mother

- When to Return to Work?
- How Long to Breastfeed?
- Whether to Express/Pump Milk?
- What Milk to Use for Missed Feedings?
- Where will Baby be Cared for?

Fertility, Sexuality, Contraception, and Breastfeeding

Fertility ———————— **Sexuality**

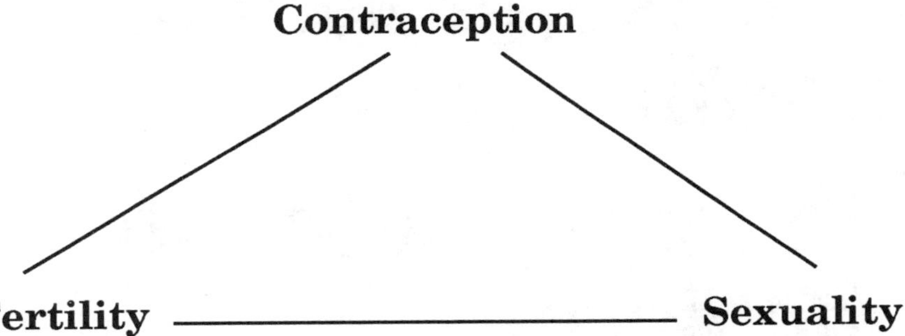

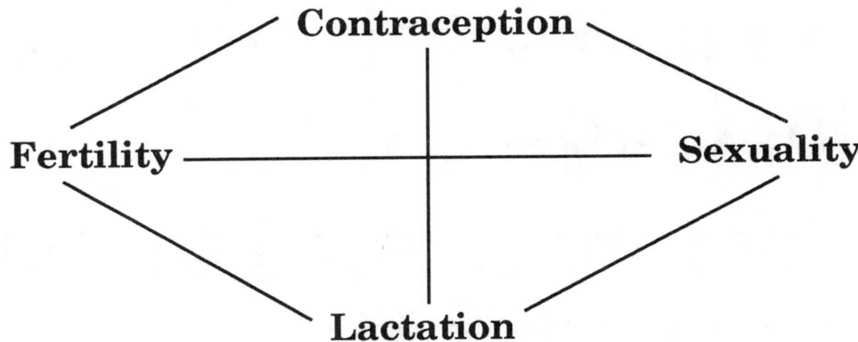

Factors Influencing Libido

- Situational factors
- Factors related to parturition
- Factors related to lactation
- Factors related to pregnancy, birth, and lactation
- Factors related to the male partner

Family Planning Options

- Condoms
- Diaphragms
- Spermicides
- Intrauterine devices (IUDs)
- Periodic abstinence (Natural Family Planning)
- Vasectomy/Tubal Ligation
- Progestin-only oral contraceptives
- Combined oral contraceptives

Physiological Mechanisms Related to Lactational Infertility

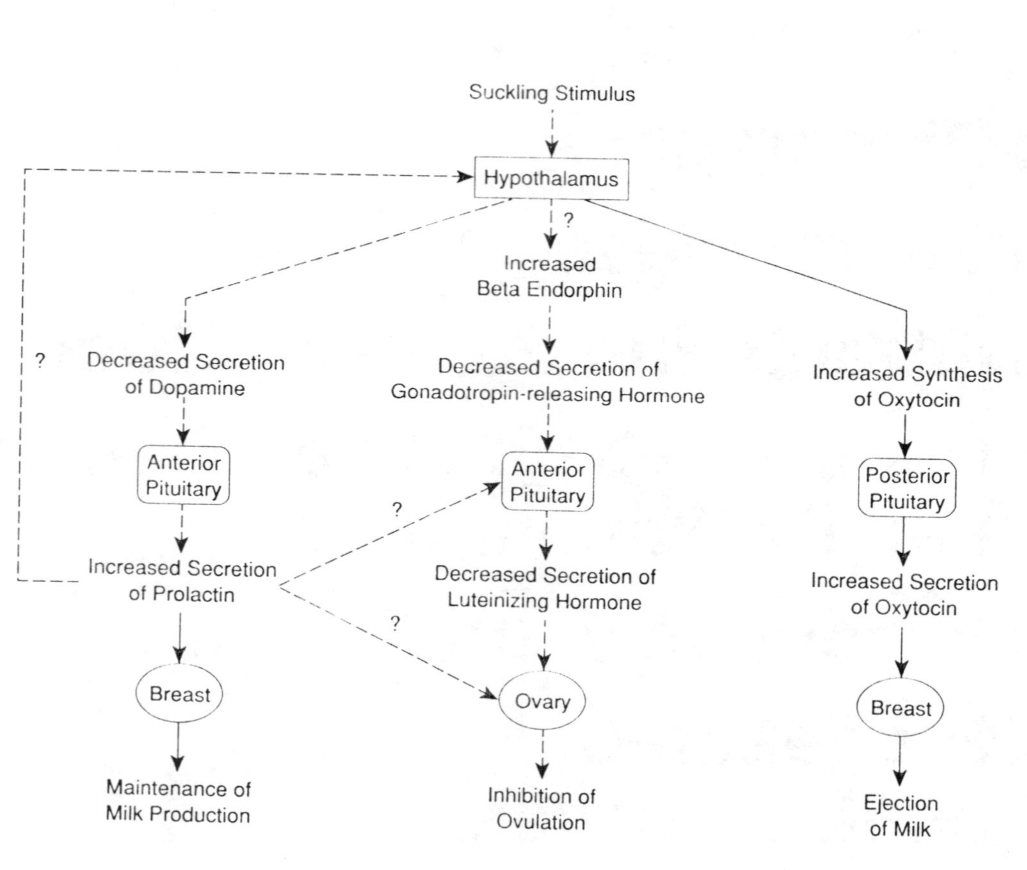

Double Protection Family Planning

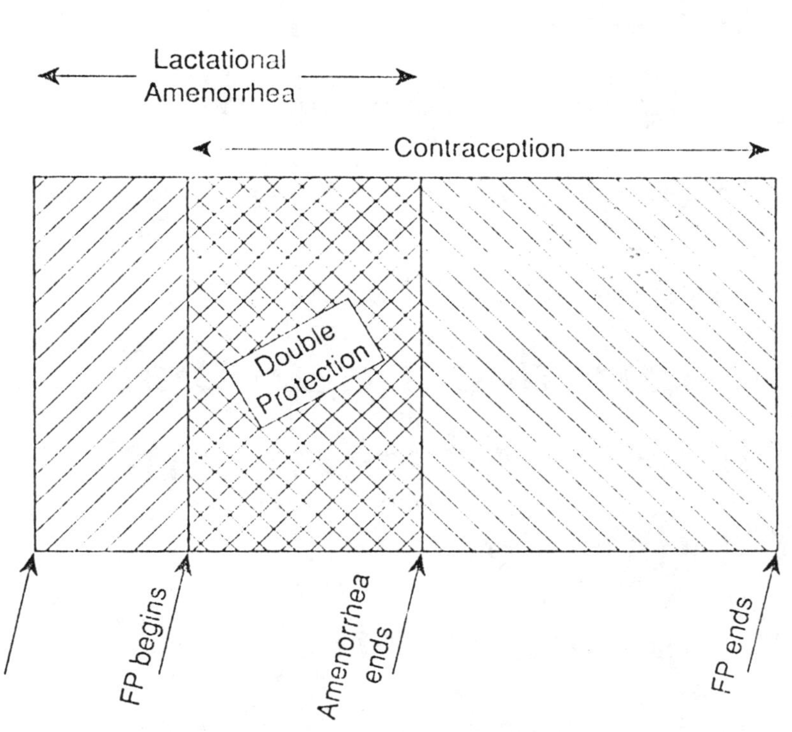

Diseases More Likely with Artificial Feeding

- Anemia
- Celiac and Crohn's disease
- Childhood lymphoma
- Gastrointestinal infection
- Infantile eczema
- Insulin-dependent diabetes
- Necrotizing enterocolitis
- Otitis media
- Respiratory infection
- Sudden infant death
- Ulcerative colitis
- Vitamin E deficiency

Breastfeeding the Ill Child

- Feedings at the breast should be continued throughout almost all illnesses if the infant is able to take oral fluids
- Assist the mother to express and store her breastmilk if the child is unable to take oral feedings
- Parents feel they are contributing to their child's welfare
- Breastfeeding confers protection against infection and promotes attachment

Chronic Sorrow

■ Loss of the "perfect" child

Stages of chronic sorrow

- Shock
- Denial
- Sadness
- Anger
- Adaptation

Congenital Heart Disease

- May not be recognized at first
- Infant suckles, pulls away to rest
- Poor weight gain, poor color
- TX: digitalis, possible surgery
- Encourage breastfeeding (it is less strenuous than bottle-feeding)
  - Feed in upright position
  - Short feedings
  - Pump milk and use feeding device, if needed

Neurologic Dysfunction

- Breastfeed if possible; feed expressed breastmilk if direct breastfeeding is not possible
- Use "C" flexed position; use front baby carrier
- Hold baby upright, flex baby's hips to feed at breast
- Skin-to-skin holding, singing, talking, cooing
- Feed drops of breastmilk in infant's mouth, stroke cheeks and tongue to stimulate

Disorganized Suckling

Infant...

- Suckles with eyes closed throughout feed
- Suckles and swallows infrequently and/or only at start of feed
- Suckle is described as weak, no strong or hurting

Mother is unable to identify swallows, or reports that they occur only briefly

Patterns of Growth Over Time (# feeds/week)

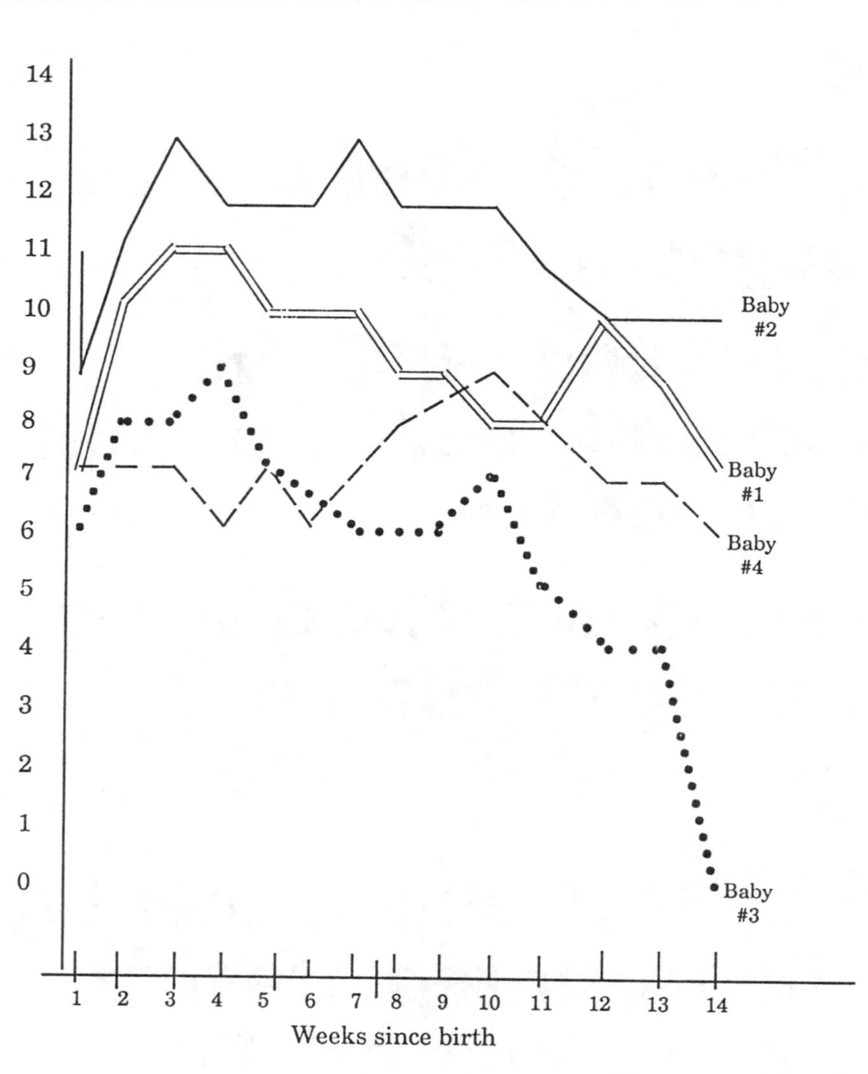

Patterns of Growth Over Time (minutes/feed/week)

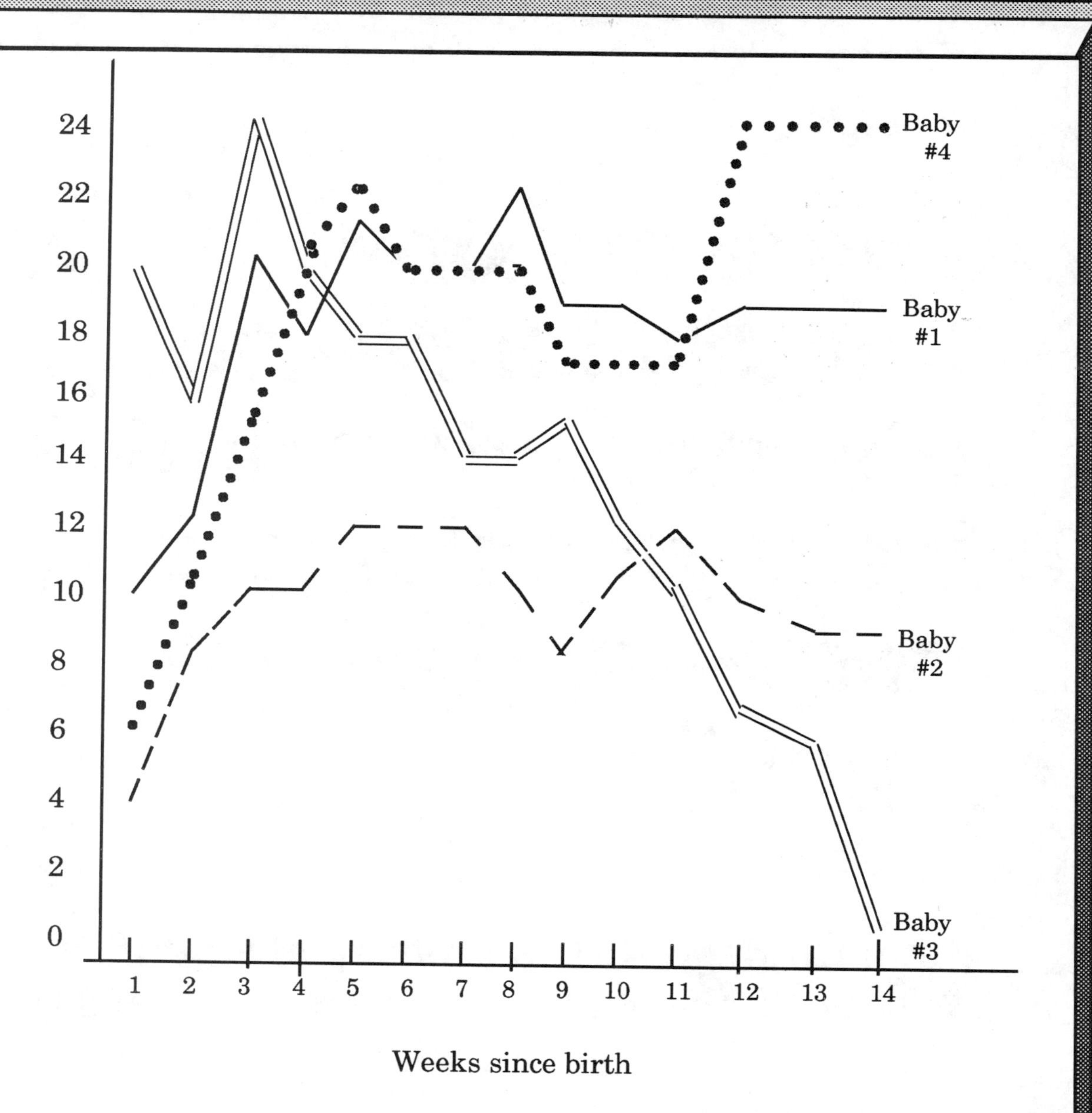

Parenting Quotation

"There are one hundred fifty-two distinctly different ways of holding a baby—and all are right."

(from Grunfeld N: *A Miscellany of Parents' Wisdom*. Philadelphia: Running Press, 1991)

Problems Relating to Slow Weight Gain

First, Rule out Organic Causes

Then, Look for...

- Mismanagement
- Disorganized Suck
- Immature CNS or Neuromuscular Disorder

The Assertive Worker...

- takes an active orientation toward work
- works constructively with others
- works collaboratively with others
- is able to give criticism and assistance
- is able to take criticism and assistance
- deals with anxiety and fear in order to continue to function effectively

Tips for Working with Women Co-Workers

- Be friendly, but do not strive to be close friends
- Be overt, not covert
- If there is a problem, confront, forget, and move on
- Communicate
- Do not make scenes or public outbursts
- Accept and love yourself
- Accept (and appreciate) that some people are not your friends, now or ever

Charts and Records

- Provide Valuable Information
- Reflect Quality of Care (quality assurance and utilization review)
- Organize Care
- Highlight Subtle Observations or Findings
- Validate Health Services for Insurance Company Reimbursement
- Provide Research Data
- Serve as Evidence in a Legal Dispute

Methods of Charting

- Narrative
- Problem-Oriented (POMA)
  - Subjective Data
  - Objective Data
  - Assessment and Nursing Diagnosis
  - Plan
  - Interventions
  - Evaluation

Legal Considerations When Providing LC Services

- Obtain permission before touching the client or her infant
- Make no promise or guarantee that will not be provided
- Avoid causing the mother, the baby, or any other member of the client's family emotional distress
- Maintain confidentiality about the mother, baby, and family

Avoid Legal Liability

- Communicate with Clients
- Document Actions
- Insure Against Liability

Solo Practice
Advantages

- Simple to Organize
- Minimal Working Capital Requirements
- Relative Freedom from Regulation
- Owner is in Direct Control
- Owner Makes all Decisions
- Tax Advantages may Apply to Small Business Owner
- All Profits go to the Owner
- Business is Easy to Dissolve

Solo Practice
Disadvantages

- Unlimited Liability
- Must Arrange for Coverage when Owner is Not Available
- Skills are Limited to those of the Solo Practitioner
- Difficulty Raising Additional Capital

Partnership
Advantages

- Easy to Organize
- Each Partner has Interest in the Business
- Greater Financial Strength
- Other Sources of Venture Capital
- Combined Managerial Skills and Judgments
- Legally Recognized Business Entity
- Possible Tax Advantages
- Limited Outside Regulation
- Business is Open when Partner has Time Off
- Ongoing Networking

Partnership
Disadvantages

- Unlimited Liability
- Lack of Authority
- Limited Authority for Decisions
- Difficulty Raising Additional Capital
- Partner Disagreements about Work Load, Income, Responsibility
- Time-off Activities Must be Coordinated

Problems Appropriate for Scientific Inquiry

- Ethical requirements can be met in all study phases
- Research design is suitable for research question
- Accessible study participants
- Study is feasible, regarding...
  - time
  - funding
  - equipment

Criteria for an Experimental Study

- Investigator controls (manipulates) treatment (independent variable)
- Experimental group receiving treatment is compared to control group not receiving treatment
- Subjects are randomly assigned to experimental and control groups

How Researchers Facilitate Clinical Practice

- Disseminate findings to clinicians
- Encourage clinicians to participate in research
- Identify clinical problems for study
- Assist clinicians in evaluating research reports

How Clinicians Facilitate Research

- Develop a questioning attitude and openness to change
- Share concerns about practice to develop pertinent clinical studies
- Critically read and evaluate research articles
- Use relevant findings in practice
- Inform other clinicians about useful study findings

Different Human Milk Preparations

- Fresh-raw Milk
- Fresh-frozen Milk
- Heat-treated Milk
- Pooled Milk

Appendix A-1

SAMPLE REPORT FOR HEALTH CARE WORKERS*

Following are elements that can be included in a report of an LC visit to the primary health care provider/referring care provider.

"This report relates to my recent visit with your patient [if going to mother's care provider]/ the mother of your patient [if going to the baby's care provider] __________ (name of patient). Below is a report of my assessment of the concerns raised.

CHIEF COMPLAINT/CONCERN:

HISTORY:

PAST MEDICAL HISTORY:

PAST SOCIAL/FAMILY HISTORY:

PHYSICAL FINDINGS/FEEDING EVALUATION:

ASSESSMENT (INCLUDING MATERNAL MILK PRODUCTION):

IMPRESSION/DIAGNOSIS:

RECOMMENDATIONS/INFORMATION SHARED WITH THE MOTHER

If you have questions about the plan outlined above, please do not hesitate to contact me. Thank you for the assistance you are providing this mother so that she might continue to breastfeed while preserving her baby's birthright to grow and thrive."

Sincerely,

[signed]

* This form may be freely copied.

Appendix A-2

DAILY FEEDING LOG*

[Use one sheet for each day of breastfeeding activity that you are recording.]

	Time Began	Time Ended	Minutes Sucking Right	Minutes Sucking Left	Audible Swallows	Output BM	Output Urine	Supplement Amount	Pumped Amount
1.									
2.									
3.									
4.									
5.									
6.									
7.									
8.									
9.									
10.									
11.									
12.									
13.									
14.									
15.									
16.									
18.									

TOTAL in 24 hours:

____ # feedings ___ #stools ____ # urine ___ # supplements

___ # pumpings ___ oz. supplements ___ oz pumped milk

* This form may be freely copied.

Appendix A-3

Daily Breastfeeding Diary

Mother's Name ____________ Health Care Provider ____________

Baby's Name ____________ Phone # ____________

Date of Birth ____________ Hospital # ____________

Sample Time	Sample; Minutes	Sample (Audible)	Sample No.Diapers	Sample Stools & Color	Sample; Suppl. Water, Formula	Sample; Amt. brstmk	Sample; Other
1 3:30 PM	Lft. 5 Rt. 10	Yes 4 No	# 2 Disposable	# 1:Yellow Liquid; small	None	None ozs	Sore Nipples

Date ______

Time of Day	Minutes of Time each Breast	Can You Hear Swallowing?	No. Wet Diapers	No. Stools & Color	Supplement[1] Amount of water/formula	Amt. Pumping[2] Breastmilk	Other
1st.	Lft. Rt.	Yes ☐ No ☐	#	#		oz.	
2nd.	Lft. Rt.	Yes ☐ No ☐	#	#		oz.	
3rd.	Lft. Rt.	Yes ☐ No ☐	#	#		oz.	
4th.	Lft. Rt.	Yes ☐ No ☐	#	#		oz.	
5th.	Lft. Rt.	Yes ☐ No ☐	#	#		oz.	
6th.	Lft. Rt.	Yes ☐ No ☐	#	#		oz.	
7th.	Lft. Rt.	Yes ☐ No ☐	#	#		oz.	
8th.	Lft. Rt.	Yes ☐ No ☐	#	#		oz.	
9th.	Lft. Rt.	Yes ☐ No ☐	#	#		oz.	
10th.	Lft. Rt.	Yes ☐ No ☐	#	#		oz.	
Totals	# of breastfeeding sessions ____	Yes No	#	#		ozs.	
Normal Range within 24 Hours	*8-10 Feeding Sessions*	*Yes*	*6-9*	*2-5*			

Date ______

Time of Day	Minutes of Time each Breast	Can You Hear Swallowing?	No. Wet Diapers	No. Stools & Color	Supplement[1] Amount of water/formula	Amt. Pumping[2] Breastmilk	Other
1st.	Lft. Rt.	Yes ☐ No ☐	#	#		oz.	
2nd.	Lft. Rt.	Yes ☐ No ☐	#	#		oz.	
3rd.	Lft. Rt.	Yes ☐ No ☐	#	#		oz.	
4th.	Lft. Rt.	Yes ☐ No ☐	#	#		oz.	
5th.	Lft. Rt.	Yes ☐ No ☐	#	#		oz.	
6th.	Lft. Rt.	Yes ☐ No ☐	#	#		oz.	
7th.	Lft. Rt.	Yes ☐ No ☐	#	#		oz.	
8th.	Lft. Rt.	Yes ☐ No ☐	#	#		oz.	
9th.	Lft. Rt.	Yes ☐ No ☐	#	#		oz.	
10th.	Lft. Rt.	Yes ☐ No ☐	#	#		oz.	
Totals	# of breastfeeding sessions ____	Yes No	#	#		ozs.	
Normal Range within 24 Hours	*8-10 Feeding Sessions*	*Yes*	*6-9*	*2-5*			

* This form may be freely copied.

Appendix A-4

MOTHER-BABY BREASTFEEDING LOG

Suggestions for Effective Breastfeeding

1. Breastfeed frequently, at least 8-10 times in 24 hours.

2. Use optimum positioning:
   a. Mother's back, shoulders, and arms are comfortably supported.
   b. Turn baby so that his/her entire body is facing you. Hold baby so that your nipple is directly in front of your baby's mouth.
   c. Support your breast 2-3 inches (5-6 cm) behind the base of the nipple.
   d. Move your breast slightly, gently stroking the baby's lower lip with your nipple. Wait for him/her to open his/her mouth WIDELY.
   e. Quickly pull the baby onto your breast.

3. Help your baby to latch on to the breast completely.
   a. Her/his lips should be flanged, and her/his nose and chin should touch your breast.
   b. Her/his tongue should be over his lower gum. (Someone else may need to check this for you.)
   c. The baby should take "a good mouthful of breast," at least one inch of breast behind the nipple.
   d. There may be jaw movement directly in front of the ear.
   e. Suckling should be strong but not painful if the baby is grasping the breast well. Let her/him suckle as long as s/he wishes. After burping and a diaper/nappy change, offer the second breast.

4. Your baby is usually getting plenty of breastmilk if these four signs are present:
   a. you see a palm-size puddle of stool <u>and</u>
   b. 6-8 wet (cloth) or 4-6 wet (paper) diapers every 24 hours <u>and</u>
   c. you hear swallows during most of each feeding, <u>and</u>
   d. your breasts feel softer after each feeding. If all four of these signs are not present, ask a lactation consultant to observe one or more feedings.

*This form may be freely copied.

Appendix A-5

SAMPLE REQUEST FOR INSURANCE COVERAGE FOR RENTAL/PURCHASE OF AN ELECTRIC BREAST PUMP*

DATE:
TO WHOM IT MAY CONCERN:
PATIENT:
NAME OF POLICY HOLDER:
POLICY NUMBER:

The following explanation of medical need is provided in order to expedite insurance coverage for the rental/purchase of an electric breast pump.

__________________________ delivered an infant(s), _______________,on _____________, and this/ these infant(s) require(s) human milk to maintain optimal health/recover from prematurity/illness.

It is well established that human milk provides optimal infant nutrition while protecting the infant against common environmental pathogens. This optimal nutrition and protection against pathogens is especially important in the first several months of the child's life. We encourage this mother to pump her breasts in order to supply her milk to her infant and to maintain lactation through the child's first several months of life.

The intermittent electric breast pump that this mother has been encouraged to rent/purchase is the most efficient, effective, and physiologic means of simulating the suckling action of a healthy human infant. A piston-style intermittent pressure electric breast pump, such as [name/brand of the pump in question] is essential for the establishment and maintenance of an adequate supply of breastmilk whenever a young child is unable to breastfeed directly.

The electric breast pump is a medical necessity, whose use is strongly encouraged, in order to support optimal, preventive health for the child named above.

Sincerely,

Physician:
Address:
City, state, ZIP/postal code:

Lactation Consultant:
Address:
City, state, ZIP/postal code:

* This form may be copied freely.

Appendix A-6

SAMPLE REQUEST FOR INSURANCE COVERAGE FOR LACTATION CONSULTATION*

DATE:
PATIENT:
NAME OF POLICY HOLDER:
POLICY NUMBER:

The following explanation of medical need is provided in order to expedite insurance coverage for lactation consulting services.

__________________ delivered an infant(s),__________________, on ______________________, and this/these infant(s) require(s) human milk to maintain optimal health/recover from prematurity/illness.

It is well established that human milk provides optimal infant nutrition while protecting the infant against common environmental pathogens. This optimal nutrition and protection against pathogens is especially important in the first year of the child's life. We encourage this mother to maintain lactation.

In my professional judgment, this mother and infant(s) need(s) the assistance of a lactation consultant for the infant to continue to be breastfed.

The cost of a lactation consultant's initial assessment, follow-up appointments (if needed), and/or the use of appropriate breastfeeding equipment is almost always LESS than the cost of one day of hospitalization.

The lactation consultation this mother has obtained, and which is detailed on the attached billing form, is assisting her to continue to breastfeed for as long as possible in order to provide optimal nutrition to her infant. I consider this service to be a valued part of comprehensive health care delivery and urge insurance coverage for these services.

Sincerely,

Physician:
Address:
City, State, ZIP/postal code:

Lactation Consultant:
Address:
City, State, ZIP/postal code:

* This form may befreely copied.

Appendix A-7

LACTATION CONSULTANT PHONE RECORD*

Call from Mother	Call from Professional
Name	Name
Address	Address
Address	Address
Age Occupation Baby's name Baby's gender Baby's date of birth Baby's current age Baby's birth weight/height Baby's current weight/height Referred by __ Ob/gyn __ Pediatrician __ Fam Pract. __ Other	Reason for referral Date/time call(s) attempted
Problem/question	
Recommendations/suggestions	
Referral to?	
Follow-up call? Follow-up visit? Date?	

*This form may be freely copied.

Appendix A-8

LACTATION CONSULTANT CONSENT FORM*

This consent form may be used as a single multi-purpose item, or separated into individualized consent forms.

__ I hereby give my consent for my lactation consultant [name] to observe me breastfeeding my infant(s) and to touch me in the course of examining my breasts and/or assessing and assisting the course of a lactation/breastfeeding episode(s) should this be necessary.

__ I hereby give my consent for my lactation consultant [name] to inform my primary physician(s) of my visit with her and of the reason(s) that prompted the visit, and/or that I have obtained/rented a breast pump in order to provide my infant(s) with my own milk in the face of barriers that might otherwise prevent me from doing so.

__ I hereby give my consent to my lactation consultant [name] to photograph me and/or my breastfeeding infant(s) for the sole purpose of assisting her in her work, including any future educational programs she might offer. I understand that my identity and the identity of my baby(ies) will be protected and that, under no circumstances, will these photographs be sold by her to any other party.

______________________________ ______________________________
Mother's signature Date

______________________________ ______________________________
Lactation consultant's signature Date

* This form may be copied freely.

Appendix A-9

SUGGESTIONS FOR ESTABLISHING A LACTATION ROOM AT THE WORKSITE*

Working mothers can continue to provide their infants with the best nutrition, breastmilk, when they return to work after childbirth. In optimal conditions, the baby would be brought to the mother's work site once or twice for feedings. Other mothers may wish to pump their breasts to provide breastmilk for subsequent feedings. With just a few provisions to facilitate the collection and storage of breastmilk, these mothers with be happier employees and will have healthier infants. A breast pumping room can be located in the health office, women's lounge or in any other small room.

A lactation program is most successful when, in addition to providing space, privacy, and appropriate equipment (i.e., hospital grade fully-automatic electric breast pumps that can be shared by several women), management is supportive and flexible. Managers need to understand the importance of mothers providing breastmilk to their babies, and that the benefits are realized by everyone, including the employer. Breastfeeding support offered in the workplace increases job productivity, employee satisfaction, and morale. The mother should be referred to community resources as needed to fulfill her breastfeeding expectations. Mothers will be most successful when the appropriate support is available.

Some mothers may choose to hand express or use their own hand-operated breast pump, milk storage containers, and small cooler. They will need only a private place to express their milk. Using a hospital grade fully-automatic electric breast pump may be more efficient for some mothers if it reduces the time the mother needs to pump her breasts.

BASIC NEEDS FOR A LACTATION ROOM

- A private area that can be locked
- A sink (or access to one) with hot and cold running water, antibacterial solution, and paper towels
- A waste basket
- A table or counter at approximately desk height for placing an electric breast pump and other supplies (A movable stand mounting for the pump is optional)
- One or more comfortable chairs that can be used next to the table where supplies are placed
- Several electrical outlets
- Disinfectant solutions for clean-up of spills (such as alcohol, diluted bleach solution, and the like)

OPTIONAL FEATURES

- A refrigerator (or nearby access) with a thermometer registering 40°F (4°C)
- One or more electric breast pumps (each mother should be required to use her own personal pump kit)
- A bulletin board for displaying baby pictures and announcements of interest to breastfeeding mothers
- A lending library of informative books or pamphlets on breastfeeding, particularly those that relate to employed breastfeeding mothers
- Referral availability of a lactation consultant for questions and concerns
- A name plate that identifies the room (examples that have been used include "Lactation Station," "Pump Room," "Expression Station")

Some employers purchase or rent one or more hospital grade electric breast pumps that can be used by several mothers. Each mother uses her own personal pumping kit which connects to the pump or hand-expresses milk into containers she has brought from home. Insulated coolers can be used to store expressed milk if a refrigerator is not available. Mothers should be instructed to wipe down the pump and other equipment on which milk has dripped after each use with a disinfectant solution. The manufacturer's instructions should be followed for suggestions pertaining to maintenance, electrical inspections, suction checks, and the like.

*This form may be freely copied.

EVALUATION FORM FOR IN-SERVICE PROGRAMS**

Teaching Breastfeeding Techniques*

Class ________________ Instructor/Facilitator________________________

Date _________________ Location __________________ Time ________

Were the objectives of the program clearly stated?
___ Yes
___ No

Were the objectives met by the program as presented?
___ Yes
___ No

Please rate (√) the following elements of this program.

	Excellent	Fair	Poor
a. As a complete educational experience	___	___	___
b. Content of the program	___	___	___
c. Organization of the program content	___	___	___
d. Teaching methods	___	___	___
e. Length/duration of program	___	___	___
f. Seqencing of program elements	___	___	___
g. Practical application of program elements	___	___	___
h. Audio-visual aids used	___	___	___
i. Environment	___	___	___
j. Speaker/presenter	___	___	___

What one task/skill did you learn from this program? ____________________

How do you plan to use that information? ___________________________

What aspect of the program did you most appreciate? ____________________

What aspect of the program most needs improvement? ___________________

Feel free to help us improve this program by offering suggestions in the space below.

* This form can serve as a model for evaluation forms of a variety of teaching modules.

** This form may be freely copied.

Sore Nipples/Severely Cracked or Damaged Nipples

Mother's name ______________________________

Infant's name ______________________ Date __________

SORE NIPPLES

Follow the instructions checked below:

❑ Apply warm wash cloths to your breasts. Massage your breasts with your fingertips.

❑ Breastfeed on your least sore breast first.

❑ Change your baby's breastfeeding positions at each feeding—cradle, clutch, side lying, etc.

❑ After feedings, rub your expressed milk into your nipples and let them air dry.

❑ Apply a thin coating of vitamin E or pure lanolin to your nipples.

❑ Expose your nipples to fresh air and sunlight.

❑ Change your cotton or paper nursing pads frequently.

❑ Wear breast shells to help the air reach your nipples. Shells also keep the fabric of your bra, blouse, or sweater from touching and irritating your sore nipples.

❑ Avoid using soap, shampoo, alcohol, or breast cream on your breasts and nipples.

❑ If soreness increases or no improvement is felt, call your lactation consultant.

SEVERELY CRACKED OR DAMAGED NIPPLES

Follow the instructions checked below:

❑ Use saline soaks (⅛ tsp. salt in 1 cup of warm water) three times a day to help clean your nipples and promote healing.

❑ Consult your health care provider about using a tiny, pinhead-sized amount of an antibiotic ointment in the crack of your nipple to promote healing and fight infection.

❑ Use a medical-grade electric breast pump ___ times per 24 hours for ___ minutes, alternating with breast massage to help empty your breasts.

❑ Breastfeed on one breast and pump the other breast.

❑ Feed your baby ___ oz. of breastmilk in 24 hours and/or ___ oz. of formula by _______ method. If formula is used as a supplement, ask your pediatrician which type of formula to feed to your baby.

❑ Keep a daily feeding diary.

❑ If redness appears on your breast or if you feel breast pain or tenderness and sudden flu-like symptoms and fever develop, call your health care provider **immediately**. These are signs of a possible breast infection that need to be medically treated.

Follow care plan for _________ days. Care plan should be used under the supervision of your primary care provider.

© 1994 Childbirth Graphics, a division of WRS Group, Inc., Waco, Texas
Developed by Nancy J. Clark, BS, IBCLC, and Josephine Tullo, BA, IBCLC

Care Provider's signature ______________________________

Follow-up date ______________ Client to call (name) ______________

Phone ______________ Follow-up visit date ______________

94375-3337-0494

*This sheet may be freely copied.

Breastfeeding Your Premature Baby

Mother's name____________________

Infant's name____________________ Date __________

HELPING YOUR BABY BEGIN BREASTFEEDING

Spend as much time as possible holding your baby's cheek against your bare breast.

If your baby seems interested in sucking, massage your breast, and express a little milk on the end of your nipple.

Hold your breast as demonstrated. Position your baby as shown.

Do not be discouraged if your baby partially opens her mouth, attempts to latch on, and falls asleep. Be patient. Babies need many practice sessions, so it may be some time before your baby is able to breastfeed well.

EACH FEEDING SESSION

Keep feeding time to approximately 20-30 minutes total.

❑ **Wake your baby** every ________ hours.

Use the following wake-up techniques:

- Undress your baby.
- Change your baby's diaper.
- Hold your baby skin to skin.
- Do baby sit-ups.
- Rub your baby's hands, feet, legs, etc.
- Massage or stroke your baby's cheeks, lips, and mouth.
- Wipe your baby's face with a warm washcloth.
- Call your baby's name or sing to your baby.

Follow care plan for ________ days. Care plan should be used under the supervision of your primary care provider.

© 1994 Childbirth Graphics, a division of WRS Group, Inc., Waco, Texas
Developed by Nancy J. Clark, BS, IBCLC, and Josephine Tullo, BA, IBCLC

DAILY FEEDING INSTRUCTIONS

In 24 hours:

Breastfeed ___ times for ___ minutes

Supplement ______ times

- amt. each feed ______ cc/oz
- total amount ______ cc/oz

______ times in 24 hours

Formula type ____________

Breastmilk ____________

Other ____________

Supplement by:
❑ Feeding tube
❑ Spoon
❑ Bottle
❑ Cup
❑ P-syringe

EACH FEEDING SESSION

Follow the feeding option checked below:

❑ **Breastfeed** for _____ minutes at each breast.

❑ **Breastfeed while using supplementation.**

❑ **Breastfeed first**, then supplement.

❑ **Prefeed your baby** _____ cc/oz before breastfeeding.

❑ **Pump your breasts** for ________ minutes using a medical-grade electric pump. Stop frequently during the pumping session to massage breasts. This will help increase the frequency of your milk ejection reflexes (let down) and your milk volume.

❑ **Label, date,** and **refrigerate** your breastmilk for future feedings.

❑ **Keep a feeding diary** according to your care provider's instructions.

❑ Have weight checks __________ at your pediatrician's office.

RECOGNIZE EFFECTIVE FEEDING

- Your baby is awake for most of the feeding.
- Your baby is positioned properly and latched onto the breast with correct mouth position as shown.
- You see movement in your baby's jaws, temples, and throat. You hear swallows as your baby feeds.
- Your baby's sucking may be rapid at first, followed by "gulps" and pauses. Rub and stimulate your baby any time the pauses are longer than five seconds.
- You should feel a drawing on your nipple and see movement in your areola.
- Your baby is content after feeding and not fussy and tense.
- Your baby has 6-8 wet diapers and at least 2 bowel movements in 24 hours. If your baby's diaper count is low, call your health care provider immediately.

Care Provider's signature____________________

Follow-up date ____________ Client to call (name)____________

Phone____________ Follow-up visit date____________

94372-3308-0494

*This sheet may be freely copied.

Suggestions for the Employed Breastfeeding Mother

BEFORE RETURNING TO WORK

• **Rest, relax, and enjoy your baby.** Try to remain at home for 6-8 weeks postpartum to recover from childbirth, to adjust to motherhood, and to establish a good milk supply. Babies often go through spurts or "frequency days" at 6 weeks, feeding more often. These spurts stimulate your breasts and ensure an abundant milk supply for the coming months.

• **Return to work on a Thursday or Friday.** This will enable you to practice and adjust your schedule and you will be less tired. Arrange to take off one day during the first month back, preferably a three-day weekend.

• **Try to locate a caregiver close to your workplace** so that you can breastfeed your baby during a lunch break and eliminate a pumping session.

• **Choose a breastpump that is time efficient and easy to use at work.** Become familiar with it and its use. Visualize your workplace. Where can you pump? How long will a pumping take to provide enough breastmilk for your baby's needs? It is best to use a medical-grade electric breastpump with a bilateral pump kit for 10-15 minutes every 3-4 hours. Alternate pumping with breast massage.

• **Two weeks prior to your return to work, begin to stockpile your breastmilk.** After morning feedings, pump some extra milk and store it in a clean plastic container or plastic bag. Label and date the container, noting any medications you have taken. Then freeze it in the coldest part of your freezer, not on the door, (see *"Handling and Storage of Breastmilk"*).

• **As a guideline for determining the total amount of milk your baby needs** in 24 hours, multiply your baby's current weight by 2.5. Then divide this total by the number of feedings your baby takes in 24 hours. This number will tell you the number of ounces your baby needs per feeding.

• **Reassess your wardrobe.** Printed blouses, sweaters, and jackets help conceal any leaking. Keep an extra blouse and bra at work along with extra nursing pads. Remember, gentle but firm pressure that presses your nipple back into your breast (fold arms) will suppress your milk ejection reflex (let down).

• **Introducing a bottle to your baby:** Warm 1-2 oz. of breastmilk in a small 4-oz. bottle with a rubber orthodontic nipple. Hold your baby in a semi-upright position, tickle your baby's lips with the bottle nipple to encourage her to open her mouth. Compress the "areola" portion (back of the bottle nipple) and put the bottle nipple in your baby's mouth, gliding it along the roof of her mouth. Speak softly and encouragingly to your baby. Tell your baby that this is a new sensation. Remember that sucking on a bottle has a new nipple taste and feels very different than sucking on a breast.

• **Some mothers find it easier if an experienced adult bottlefeeder or father introduces the bottle.** Babies who are reluctant to bottlefeed need lots of gentle, non-threatening exposure to rubber nipples. Let them play with the bottle when they are not hungry. Some babies never take a bottle and can be spoonfed or cup fed with a sipper cup.

• **When introducing your baby to her caregiver, do so gradually.** On the first day, breastfeed your baby before leaving. Return within 1-2 hours. Before leaving, breastfeed at the caregiver's if possible. On the next day, extend the length of time you are gone and have the caregiver feed your baby a bottle of breastmilk. Gradually over several days, extend the length of time that the baby is left with the caregiver. Your baby will soon learn that the caregiver feeds her in one way in this setting and that mother breastfeeds her in a home setting. Any milk pumped at your work site can be fed to your baby the next day. Check with your baby's pediatrician before using any formula supplementation.

• **The night before you return to work, pack your diaper bag and pump kit.** Secure the car seat in your car. Select clothes for the next day. Pack your pump, lunch, drinks, and nutritious snacks. Place freezer packs for your milk storage cooler in the freezer and go to bed early.

If you have any questions about this information, please contact your health care provider.

© 1994 Childbirth Graphics, a division of WRS Group, Inc., Waco, Texas
Developed by Nancy J. Clark, BS, IBCLC, and Josephine Tullo, BA, IBCLC

Printed on recycled paper

94373-3305-0494

* This sheet may be freely copied.

Suggestions for the Employed Breastfeeding Mother (cont.)

DAILY ROUTINE

• **Establish a relaxed morning routine.** Make time to breastfeed before you get ready for work. Breastfeeding your baby before leaving the house is ideal. You may bring your baby to bed with you to breastfeed an hour before getting up or you may want to breastfeed your baby prior to leaving her with your caregiver.

PUMPING & FACILITATING YOUR MILK EJECTION REFLEX (LETDOWN)

• **If you and your baby are separated for 8-10 hours,** you will need to pump 3-4 times to provide a full supply of breastmilk and stimulate your breasts adequately. For a 4-6 hour separation, you will need two pumpings.

• **Ten to fifteen minutes prior to a pumping,** try to eat and drink something and begin to unwind. Do some shoulder exercises and neck rolls to release tension in your upper body. Assemble your pump kit. Massage your breasts while thinking of your baby and do some deep breathing. Follow the instructions for pumping in your pump kit. Remember, you are pumping for comfort and for breast stimulation to maintain your future milk supply.

• **If you experience a decrease in your milk supply:**

- drink more fluids
- try to get more rest
- add additional pumpings to your day

Additional pumpings could be done after your baby breastfeeds.

• **Combining work and breastfeeding** takes organization and commitment, but the rewards are tremendous to mother, father, and baby. Eat regular meals and rest as much as possible. Get help with housework and spend those first few weeks at home recovering from childbirth, establishing your milk supply, and enjoying your baby. Set aside special time for skin-to-skin cuddling and relax with your baby. After you return to work, breastfeed your baby as much as possible in the evenings and on weekends. Your baby is the "best breastpump" to maintain your supply. If you have any concerns, call a breastfeeding counselor or lactation consultant for support and help.

If you have any questions about this information, please contact your health care provider.

© 1994 Childbirth Graphics, a division of WRS Group, Inc., Waco, Texas
Developed by Nancy J. Clark, BS, IBCLC, and Josephine Tullo, BA, IBCLC

Printed on recycled paper

94373-3305-0494

Handling and Storage of Breastmilk:
Suggestions for a Healthy Mother and a Healthy Baby

PREPARING TO STORE YOUR BREASTMILK

Before pumping your breastmilk always wash your hands. Be sure to use a clean breastpump. Breastmilk containers should be clean, dry, and capped. Use a separate container for each pumping or use specially designed plastic bags to hold your breastmilk. Label each bottle with the date, any medications, or unusual foods you ate. Use your breastmilk in the order you pumped and stored it. It is normal for the color and consistency of breastmilk to vary from mother to mother. Shake stored breastmilk gently before using.

FRESH BREASTMILK

Fresh breastmilk is more stable than formula. Frozen breastmilk is fragile and less stable than formula.

Refrigerate pumped breastmilk immediately in your refrigerator or cooler.

Always transport your breastmilk in an insulated carrying case with ice packs. This cooler should cool below 44° Fahrenheit.

STORING FRESH BREASTMILK

Fresh breastmilk may be stored in the refrigerator for 48 hours. You may freeze your breastmilk if it has been refrigerated no longer than 48 hours. Do not freeze breastmilk that has been refrigerated longer than 48 hours.

HANDLING FRESH BREASTMILK

Do not microwave or boil breastmilk.

Warm your refrigerated breastmilk under running tap water. Slowly increase the heat of the water in order to heat your breastmilk.

Feed your baby right away after you have heated the milk to its desired temperature. Any unused portion of this milk may be refrigerated and used at the next feeding (within 4–6 hours). Do not add more milk to this bottle or save it for more than 6 hours. If you have used a bottle, remove the nipple and seal the bottle or bag before storing.

FROZEN BREASTMILK

To add more milk to some that is already frozen, chill it first in the refrigerator for at least 30 minutes. This prevents the top layer of frozen milk from defrosting as you add the new breastmilk.

STORING FROZEN BREASTMILK

You may store your breastmilk for:

- 1 month in a separate compartment freezer that does not reach at least 0° Fahrenheit. This milk should be insulated from the defrost cycle. Do not store milk inside the freezer door. If your freezer keeps ice cream rock hard, you may freeze your breastmilk for up to 6 months.
- 6 months in a freezer 0° Fahrenheit or below.
- 6 months in a deep freezer if the milk is insulated from the defrost cycle.

THAWING FROZEN BREASTMILK

Do not microwave or boil breastmilk.

Thaw breastmilk under running tap water. Slowly increase the heat of the water in order to heat the breastmilk.Thawing frozen breastmilk slowly in the refrigerator may allow bacterial growth (pathogens) and is not recommended.

Primary Reference: Riordan, J., Auerbach, K. Breastfeeding and Human Lactation, Jones & Bartlett Publishers, Boston, 1993.

If you have any questions about this information, please contact your health care provider.

© 1994 Childbirth Graphics, a division of WRS Group, Inc., Waco, Texas
Developed by Nancy J. Clark, BS, IBCLC, and Josephine Tullo, BA, IBCLC

Printed on recycled paper

94376-3306-0494

*This sheet may be freely copied.

LA LECHE LEAGUE INTERNATIONAL
1400 North Meacham Road • Schaumburg, IL 60173 USA • 708.519.7730 • fax 708.519.0035 • 1.800.LA LECHE

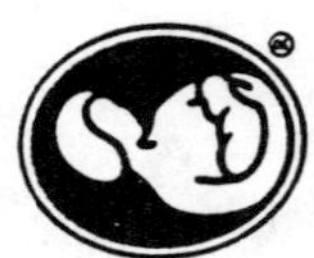

How To Know Your Healthy Full-Term Breastfed Baby Is Getting Enough Milk

- Your baby may have only one or two wet diapers during the first day or two after birth. Beginning about the third or fourth day, your baby will have at least six to eight really wet cloth diapers (five to six disposables).
- Your baby will pass meconium, the greenish-black, tarry first stool, over the first day or two. Baby will begin having at least two to five bowel movements a day beginning about the third day after birth.
- Your baby may lose up to ten percent of his/her birth weight during the first three or four days. Once your milk supply becomes more plentiful on the third or fourth day, expect your baby to begin gaining at least four to seven ounces (113 to 198 grams) per week or at least a pound (454 grams) a month. Be sure to count weight gain from the lowest weight (his weight on the third or fourth day), not from birth weight.
- Your baby will nurse frequently, often every one and one-half to three hours, averaging about eight to twelve times a day.
- Your baby will appear healthy, his color will be good, his skin will be firm, he will be filling out and growing in length and head circumference, and he will be alert and active.

If You Need To Increase Your Milk Supply

GET HELP. If your baby is not gaining well, or is losing weight, keep in close touch with your baby's doctor. In many cases, improved breastfeeding techniques will quickly resolve the situation, but in some cases, slow weight gain may indicate a serious health problem.

NURSE FREQUENTLY for as long as your baby will nurse. A sleepy baby may need to be awakened and encouraged to nurse more frequently.

OFFER BOTH BREASTS AT EACH FEEDING. This will ensure that your baby gets all the milk available and that both breasts are stimulated frequently.

BE SURE THAT BABY IS POSITIONED CORRECTLY AT THE BREAST. Baby's lips should be on the areola (dark area surrounding the nipple), well behind the nipple. If you are not sure baby is sucking well, or feel any soreness, ask your health care provider, La Leche League Leader, or other breastfeeding specialist to help you.

TRY SWITCH NURSING. Switching breasts two or three times throughout each feeding will help to keep your baby interested in nursing. Switch breasts as soon as baby's sucking slows down and he swallows less often. Your milk supply will be stimulated by using both breasts at least twice at each feeding.

GIVE YOUR BABY ONLY BREAST MILK. If your baby has been receiving formula supplements, do not cut these out abruptly. Gradually cut back on the amount of supplement as your milk supply increases, but watch baby's wet and soiled diapers to be sure he is getting enough milk. Stay in touch with your baby's doctor.

ALL YOUR BABY'S SUCKING SHOULD BE AT THE BREAST. If some supplement is necessary temporarily, it can be given by spoon, cup, or with a nursing supplementer, a device used to feed baby additional milk through a small tube while he nurses at the breast.

PAY ATTENTION TO YOUR OWN NEED FOR REST, RELAXATION, PROPER DIET, AND SUFFICIENT FLUIDS. Taking care of yourself will aid in increasing your milk supply and improving your general sense of well-being.

If you have any further questions or concerns be sure to get in touch with your La Leche League Leader or other breastfeeding specialist. Remember that a baby who is not gaining weight will need to be checked regularly by the doctor.

© 1995 La Leche League International

No.457 December 1994

* This sheet may be freely copied.

BREASTFEEDING

EARLY START

- Put baby to the breast to nurse as soon as possible after birth.

LATCHING ON

- Sit back comfortably (don't lean over baby)
- Place baby's head in crook of elbow. Pull baby's feet in close to other side. Hold baby at level of breast. BABY'S FACE AND BODY ARE TURNED TOWARDS MOTHER.

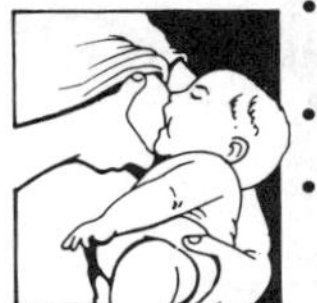

- Tickle middle of baby's lower lip, wait for him to open WIDE.
- Pull baby closer when ready to latch on.
- Make sure that a large part of areola is drawn in.

COLOSTRUM

- Produced in first few days.
- Small in quantity (teaspoons, not ounces).
- Protects against infection.
- Clears meconium — Helps prevent jaundice.
- Satisfies baby's thirst and hunger.

> Frequent breastfeeding stimulates milk production. It is not true that resting the breasts results in more milk.

WHY NO BOTTLE?

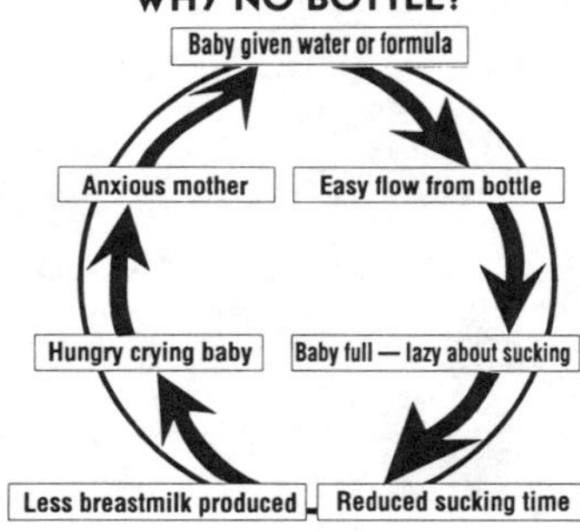

BABY NEEDS NIGHT FEEDINGS

Easily digested breastmilk passes quickly through the digestive system. This is why breastfed babies wake at night.

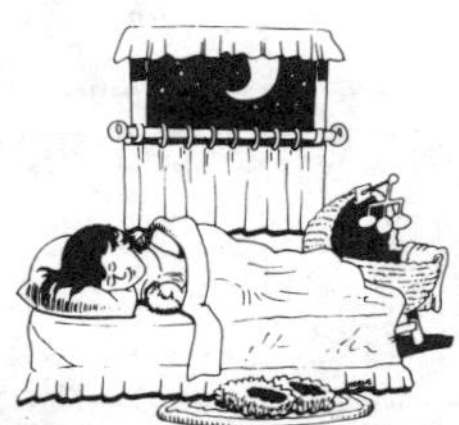

HOW OFTEN?

Baby needs to nurse 10-14 times in 24 hours. The more you nurse, the more milk you will have.

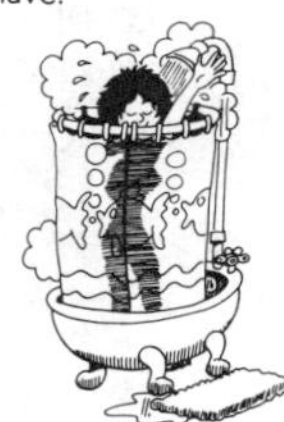

ENGORGEMENT

- Warm showers or compresses before feeding
- Soften breast by expressing some milk
- Nurse often!

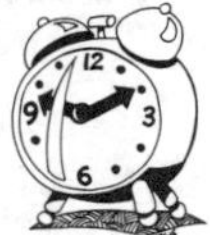

WATCH YOUR BABY... NOT THE CLOCK!

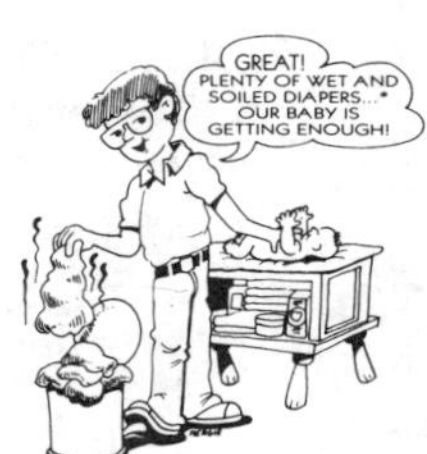

ENOUGH MILK?

*After the milk comes in ...
6-8 wet diapers
3-5 bowel movements per day means baby is getting enough breastmilk.

MILK TOO WEAK?

Never! Milk changes throughout the feeding. Express one drop of milk before and after a feeding and see the difference. Foremilk is watery to satisfy thirst. Hindmilk is creamy to satisfy hunger.

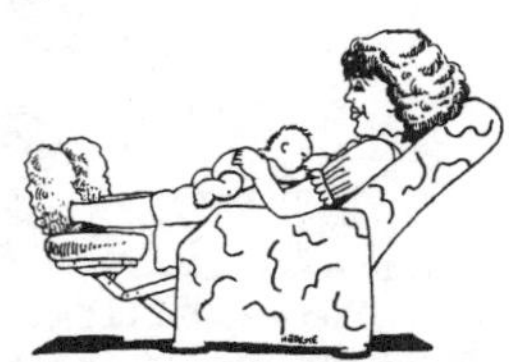

TOO MUCH MILK

- Offer one breast at a feeding.
- Offer the same breast if baby wants more soon after a feeding.
- Feeding against gravity may slow the flow.

SORE NIPPLES

> REMEMBER: Correct positioning is most important for preventing sore nipples.

- Break suction before taking baby off the breast.
- Give shorter, more frequent feedings.
- Offer the least sore breast first.
- Avoid plastic against nipples.
- Use only water for washing.
- Expose to sun & air as much as possible.

BLOCKED DUCT

If milk becomes blocked a tender lump may appear in the breast.

- Apply heat
- Get plenty of rest
- Nurse frequently
- Check positioning

GROWTH SPURTS

Baby may nurse more often at times to build milk supply. "Frequency days" often occur around 3 weeks of age.

OLDER BABY — SOFTER BREAST

When the milk supply is established, breasts get softer naturally.

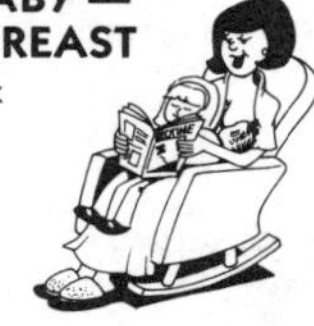

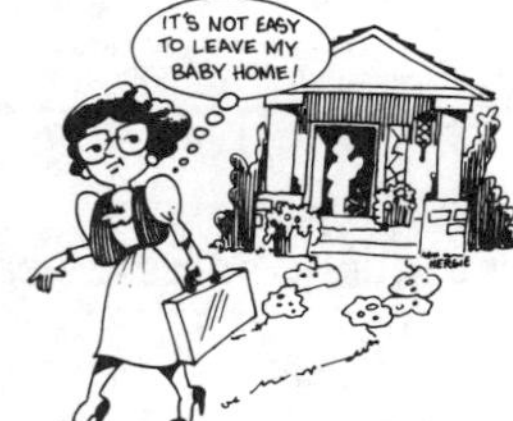

BACK TO WORK

- Find out about facilities at work for expressing and storing breastmilk.
- Start working only when milk supply is well-established.
- Feed as often as possible when at home.

CHOICES

Breastmilk Only	Breast and Bottle
Express and store milk at work in a refrigerator.	Express milk to feel comfortable and to stimulate lactation while at work.
Take milk home for the next day's feeds.	Use breastmilk substitutes when at work.
Frequent breastfeeding when at home.	Breastfeed when at home.

SPONSORED BY

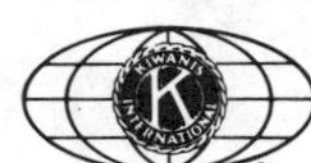

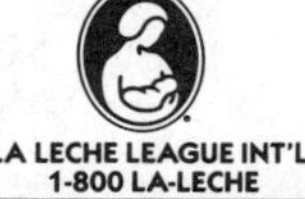

LA LECHE LEAGUE INT'L.
1-800 LA-LECHE

• The page may be freely copied.

¡¡Lea esto!! Es importante para la vida de su bebé.

DANDO EL PECHO

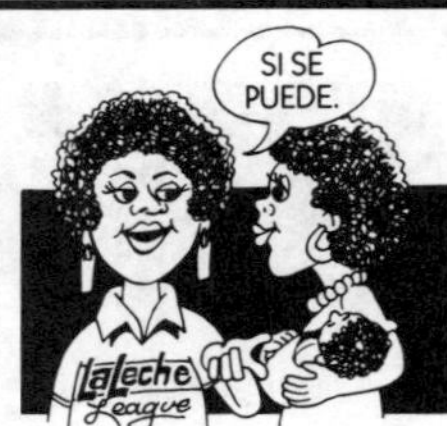

SI SE PUEDE.

COMIENCE CUANTO ANTES

- Dele el pecho tan pronto como sea posible despues del parto.

PONIENDOLO AL PECHO

- Sientese con la espalda comoda (no se incline sobre el bebé).
- Ponga la cabeza del bebé en el doblez del codo.
- Arrimese los pies del bebé cerca del otro lado. Abrace al bebé al nivel del pecho. LA CARA Y EL CUERPO DEL BEBÉ VOLTEADOS HACIA LA MADRE.

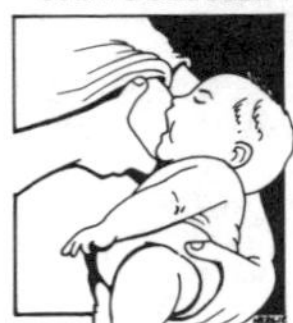

- Toque el labio inferior, espere a que abra bién la boca.
- Arrimese al bebé más cerca cuando esté listo para agarrarlo.
- Asegurese que el bebé tenga la mayor parte de la areola dentro de la boca.

EL CALOSTRO

- Se produce en los primeros dias.
- Poca cantidad (cucharaditas, no onzas.)
- Protege contra infecciones.
- Expulsa el meconio — Ayuda a prevenir la ictericia.
- Satisface el hambre y la sed del bebé.

> Mientras más dé el pecho, más leche produce. No es cierto que dejando descansar el pecho resulta en más leche.

¿PORQUE NO DARLE EL BIBERON?

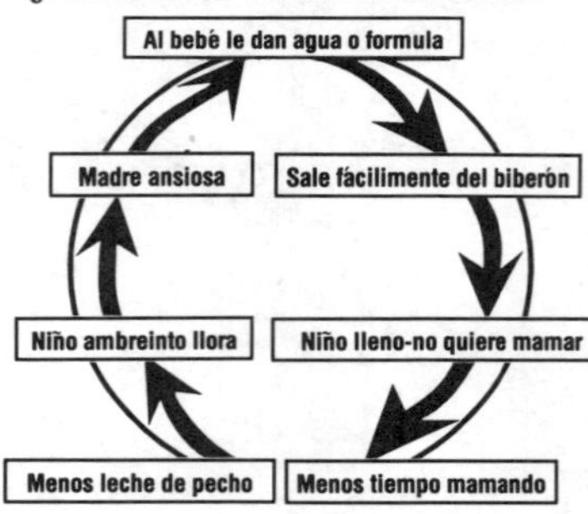

Al bebé le dan agua o formula
Sale fácilmente del biberòn
Niño lleno-no quiere mamar
Menos tiempo mamando
Menos leche de pecho
Niño ambreinto llora
Madre ansiosa

EL BEBÉ NECESITA MAMAR DE NOCHE

La leche materna se digiere facilmente y pasa rapidamente por el sistema digestivo. Por eso los bebés despiertan de noche.

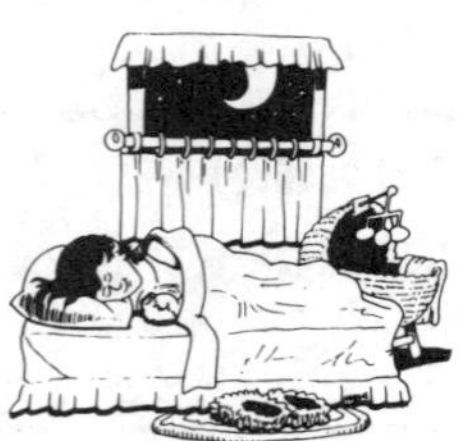

¿QUE TAN SEGUIDO?

El bebé necesita mamar 10 o 12 veces en 24 horas. Mientras más mame, más leche tendra Ud.

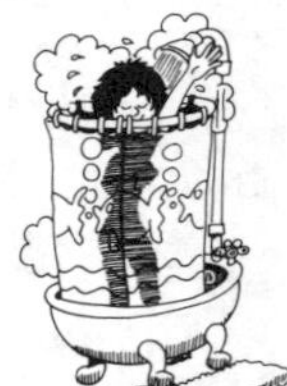

PLÉTORA

- Baños de regadera calientes o fomentos antes de dar el pecho.
- Ablande el pecho sacandose le leche.
- Dele el pecho muy seguido.

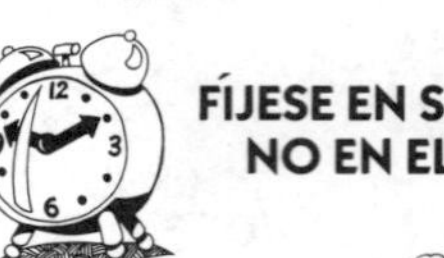

FÍJESE EN SU BEBÉ ... NO EN EL RELOJ

¡QUE BIEN!
Muchos pañales mojados y sucios está tomando suficiente leche.

¿SUFICIENTE LECHE?

*Despues de que baja la leche
5-8 pañales mojados
3-5 pañales sucios
por día indican que el bebé está tomado suficiente leche.

¿LECHE MUY AGUADA?

¡Nunca! La leche cambia en las tetadas. Saquese una gota de leche antes y después de la tetada y verá la diferencia. La primera leche tiene mucha aqua para satisfacer la sed. La leche despues es cremosa para satisfacer la hambre.

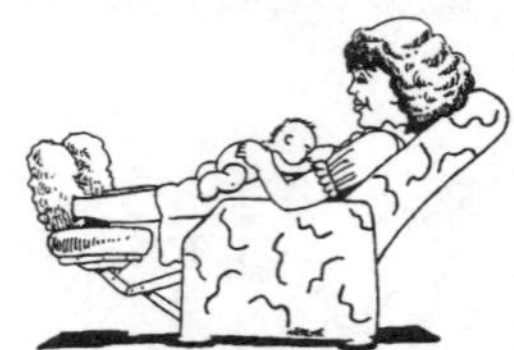

DEMASIADA LECHE

- Ofrenca un pecho en cada comida.
- Ofrenca el mismo pecho si el bebé quiere más lugeo después de mamar.
- Mamar contra la gravedad puede disminuir el flujo.

PEZONES ADOLORIDOS

> RECUERDE: La posición correcta es muy importante para evitar pezones adoloridos.

- Rompa la succión antes de quitar al bebé del pecho.
- Las tetadas deben ser más cortas y frequentes.
- Ofrezca primero el pecho menos adolorido.
- No use plástico en los pezones.
- Use sólo agua para lavarlos.
- Pongalos al sol y al aire lo más que pueda.

DUCTO BLOQUEADO

Si la leche se bloquea puede aparecerle hinchazón y dolor.

- Aplique calor.
- Dejelo mamar más seguido.
- Descanse.
- Acomodese bién al bebé.

ETAPAS DE CRECIMIENTO

El bebé puede mamar más seguido para aumentar la producción de leche. Los dias de "más frequencia" ocurren alrededor de las tres semanas de edad.

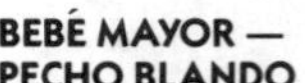

BEBÉ MAYOR — PECHO BLANDO

Cuando la producción de leche se ha establecido, el pecho se vuelve más blando.

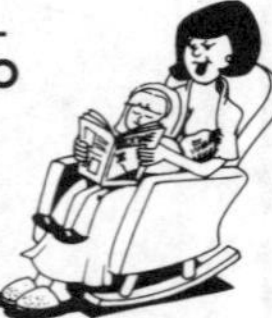

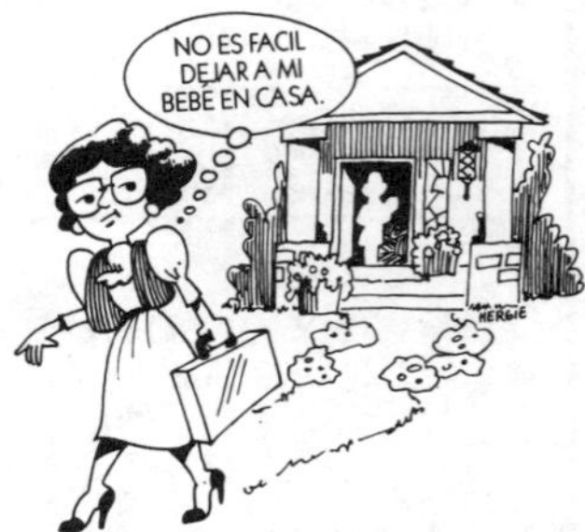

NO ES FACIL DEJAR A MI BEBE EN CASA.

DE REGRESO AL TRABAJO

- Pregunte si hay donde sacarse y guardar la leche.
- No empieze a trabajar hasta que ya esté establecida la leche.
- Cundo esté en casa, dele el pecho al bebé lo más que pueda.

OPCIONES

Leche de Pecho	Pecho y Biberón
Saquese y guarde la leche en el refrigerador. Lleve la leche a casa para la comida del dia siguiente. Dele el pecho seguido en casa.	Saquese la leche para sentirse mejor y estimular la lactancia. Use sustitutos de leche cuando trabaje. Dé el pecho en casa seguido.

PATROCINADO POR

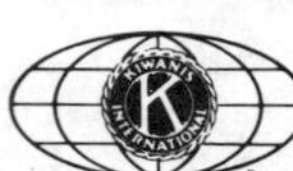

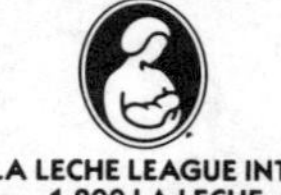

LA LECHE LEAGUE INT'L.
1-800 LA-LECHE

• Esta página puede reproducirse sin restricciones.

SAMPLE PATIENT INSTRUCTIONS*

In different settings, checklists of information/instructions can be useful. Following are samples of such checklists.

ENGORGEMENT

__ Moist heat prior to breastfeeding
__ Breast massage
__ Breastfeed frequently; _____x24 hrs
__ Cold compresses after breastfeeding
__ Hand expression
__ Express/pump breasts every ____ hrs
__ Slow breathing/relaxation exercises
__ Follow up on __________________
(date)
  __ by phone
  __ by home visit
  __ by office visit

MASTITIS

__ Moist heat prior to breastfeeding
__ Gentle breast massage
__ Breastfeed affected breast first
__ Bedrest for 24 hours
__ Pain medication, as prescribed
__ Antibiotic _______x _______
__ Breastfeed frquently; ____x24 hrs
__ Follow up on ______________
(date)
  __ by phone
  __ by home visit
  __ by office visit

SORE NIPPLES

__ Check positioning; improve if necessary
__ Check latch-on; improve if necessary
__ Breastfeed frequently; _____x24 hrs
__ Cold/ice to nipple before breastfeeding
__ Lanolin after each breastfeeding
__ (if cracks/fissures, hydrogen peroxide to nipples after each breastfeeding
__ Slow breathing/relaxation exercises
__ Follow up on __________________
(date)
  __ by phone
  __ by home visit
  __ by office visit

THRUSH

__ Medication for nipples after each breastfeeding for ____ days (OTC)
__ Medication for baby's mouth after each feeding x ___ as prescribed
__ Boil all rubber teats, pacifiers/ dummies/teethers daily; discard after 7 days
__ If vaginal yeast infection, treat
__ Express/pump if breastfeeding too painful; ___hrs x ___ days
__ See checklist for sore nipples
__ Follow up on ______________
(date)
  __ by phone
  __ by home visit
  __ by office visit

*This form may be freely copied.

Hospital Self-Appraisal Tool for the UNICEF Baby-Friendly Hospital Initiative*

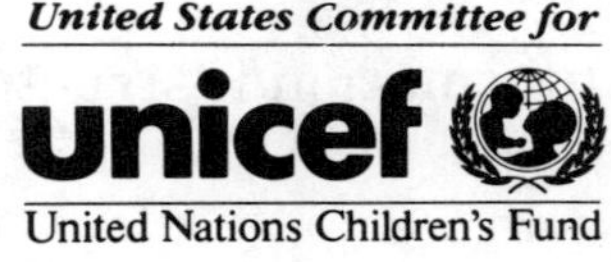

Using the Hospital Self Appraisal Tool to Review Policies and Practices

Any hospital or health facility that is interested in receiving a Certificate of Intent to Support the Principles of the Global Baby-Friendly Hospital Initiative should—as a first step—appraise its current practices in relation to the Ten Steps to Successful Breastfeeding.

The checklist that follows will permit a hospital, birthing center, or other health facility giving maternity care to make a quick initial appraisal or review of its practices in support of breastfeeding. Completion of this initial self-review form is the first stage of the process of meeting the requirements to receive a Certificate of Intent from the U.S. Committee for UNICEF. (In the United States, the baby-friendly designation process is still being developed; final recommendations will be issued in 1994.)

Hospitals are encouraged to bring their key management and clinical staff together to review the Self Appraisal Tool and develop a plan of action based on the results of the self appraisal. Suggestions for specific action for an in-house group of hospital management and clinical staff are to establish 1) a written breastfeeding policy, 2) a written curriculum for any training in lactation management given to hospital staff caring for mothers and babies, 3) a written outline of the content to be covered in antenatal health education about breastfeeding. Existence of such written documents provides evidence of on-going institutional commitment to breastfeeding and ensures continued promotion even with changes in staff. Consultation with the U.S. Committee for UNICEF can provide more information on policies and training that will contribute to increasing the Baby-Friendliness of health facilities.

For more information contact:
Minda Lazarov
U.S. Committee for UNICEF
615-322-2470

* This multi-page document may be freely copied.

OSPITAL DATA SHEET Date ______________, 19 _____

no nursery for normal well newborns exists, write "none" in space provided.

ospital Name: ____

ddress: ____

ity, District, or Region: ______________________ Country: ______________________

ame of Chief Hospital Administrator: ______________________ Telephone: ______________________

ames of senior Nursing Officers (or other personnel in charge):

For the Facility: ______________________ Telephone: ______________________

For the Maternity Ward:______________________ Telephone: ______________________

For the Antenatal Service: ______________________ Telephone:______________________

Name of person to be contacted for additional information: ______________________

ype of Hospital: Government Private - Not for profit Private - For profit

Mission Teaching Other: ______________________

OSPITAL CENSUS DATA:

otal bed capacity: ________________

_____ in labour and delivery area

_____ in the maternity ward

_____ in the normal nursery

_____ in the special care nursery

_____ in other areas for mothers and children

otal Deliveries in year 199___:_____

_____ were by Caesarean Caesarean rate __________%

_____ were low birth weight babies (<2500g) Low birth weight rate __________%

_____ were in special care Special care rate __________%

nfant feeding data for deliveries from records or staff reports:

_____ mother /infant pairs discharged in the past month

_____ mother/infant pairs breastfeeding at discharge in the past month __________%

_____ mother/infant pairs breastfeeding exclusively from birth to discharge in the past month __________%

_____ infants discharged in the past month who have received at least one bottlefeed since birth __________%

ow was the infant feeding data obtained?

_____ From records

_____ Percentages are an estimate, provided by: ______________________

lame of person(s) filling out this form:

____

____

STEP 1. Have a written breastfeeding policy that is routinely communicated to all health care sta

1.1 Does the health facility have an explicit written policy for protecting, promoting, and supporting breastfeeding that addresses all 10 steps to successful breastfeeding in maternity services . . . . Yes ☐ No ☐

1.2 Does the policy protect breastfeeding by prohibiting all promotion of and group instruction for using breastmilk substitutes, feeding bottles and teats? . . . . Yes ☐ No ☐

1.3 Is the breastfeeding policy available so all staff who take care of mothers and babies can refer to it? . . . . Yes ☐ No ☐

1.4 Is the breastfeeding policy posted or displayed in all areas of the health facility which serve mothers, infants, and/or children? . . . . Yes ☐ No ☐

1.5 Is there a mechanism for evaluating the effectiveness of the policy? . . . . Yes ☐ No ☐

STEP 2. Train all health care staff in skills necessary to implement this policy.

2.1 Are all staff aware of the advantages of breastfeeding and acquainted with the facility's policy and services to protect, promote, and support breastfeeding?. . . . . Yes ☐ No ☐

2.2 Are all staff caring for women and infants oriented to the breastfeeding policy of the hospital on their arrival?. . . . . Yes ☐ No ☐

2.3 Is training on breastfeeding and lactation management given to all staff caring for women and infants within six months of their arrival?. Yes ☐ No ☐

2.4 Does the training cover at least eight of the Ten Steps to Successful Breastfeeding? . . . . Yes ☐ No ☐

2.5 Is the training on breastfeeding and lactation management at least 18 hours in total, including a minimum of 3 hours of supervised clinical experience?. . . . . Yes ☐ No ☐

2.6 Has the healthcare facility arranged for specialized training in lactation management of specific staff members?. . . . . Yes ☐ No ☐

STEP 3. Inform all pregnant women about the benefits and management of breastfeeding.

3.1 Does the hospital include an antenatal care clinic? Or an antenatal inpatient ward?. . . . . Yes ☐ No ☐

3.2 If yes, are most pregnant women attending these antenatal services informed about the benefits and management of breastfeeding?. . . . . Yes ☐ No ☐

3.3 Do antenatal records indicate whether breastfeeding has been discussed with the pregnant woman? . . . . Yes ☐ No ☐

3.4 Is a mother's antenatal record available at the time of delivery? . . . . Yes ☐ No ☐

3.5 Are pregnant women protected from oral or written promotion of group instruction for artificial feeding? . . . . Yes ☐ No ☐

3.6 Does the healthcare facility take into account a woman's intention to breastfeed when deciding on the use of a sedative, an analgesic, or an anesthetic, (if any) during labour and delivery? . . . . Yes ☐ No ☐

3.7 Are staff familiar with the effects of such medicaments on breastfeeding? . . . . Yes ☐ No ☐

3.8 Does a woman who has never breastfed or who has previously encountered problems with breastfeeding receive special attention and support from the staff of the healthcare facility? . . . . Yes ☐ No ☐

STEP 4. Help mothers initiate breastfeeding within a half-hour of birth.

4.1 Are mothers whose deliveries are normal given their babies to hold, with skin contact, within a half-hour of completion of the second stage of labour and allowed to remain with them for at least the first hour? . . . . Yes ☐ No ☐

4.2 Are the mothers offered help by a staff member to initiate breastfeeding during this first hour? . . . . Yes ☐ No ☐

4.3 Are mothers who have had caesarean deliveries given their babies to hold, with skin contact, within a half hour after they are able to respond to their babies? . . . . Yes ☐ No ☐

4.4 Do the babies born by caesarean stay with their mothers, with skin contact, at this time for at least 30 minutes? . . . . Yes ☐ No ☐

STEP 5. Show mothers how to breastfeed and how to maintain lactation, even if they should be separated from their infants.

5.1 Does nursing staff offer all mothers further assistance with breastfeeding within six hours of delivery? . . . . Yes ☐ No ☐

5.2 Are most breastfeeding mothers able to demonstrate how to correctly position and attach their babies for breastfeeding? . . . . Yes ☐ No ☐

5.3 Are breastfeeding mothers shown how to express their milk or given information on expression and/or advised of where they can get help, should they need it? . . . . Yes ☐ No ☐

5.4 Are staff members or counselors who have specialized training in breastfeeding and lactation management available full-time to advise mothers during their stay in healthcare facilities and in preparation for discharge? . . . . Yes ☐ No ☐

5.5 Does a woman who has never breastfed or who has previously encountered problems with breastfeeding receive special attention and support from the staff of the healthcare facility? . . . . Yes ☐ No ☐

5.6 Are mothers of babies in special care helped to establish and maintain lactation by frequent expression of milk? . . . . Yes ☐ No ☐

STEP 6. Give newborn infants no food or drink other than breastmilk, unless *medically* indicated.

6.1 Do staff have a clear understanding of what the few acceptable reasons are for prescribing food or drink other than breastmilk for breastfeeding babies?. . . . . Yes ☐ No ☐

6.2 Do breastfeeding babies receive no other food or drink (than breastmilk) unless medically indicated?
Breastmilk only. . . . . Yes ☐
Some other food/drink . . . . No ☐

6.3 Are any breastmilk substitutes including special formulas which are used in the facility purchased in the same way as any other foods or medicines?. . . . . Yes ☐ No ☐

6.4 Do health facility and health care workers refuse free or low-cost* supplies of breastmilk substitutes, paying close to retail market price for any?. . . . . Yes ☐ No ☐

6.5 Is all promotion of infant foods or drinks other than breastmilk absent from the facility? . . . . Yes ☐ No ☐

STEP 7. Practice rooming-in—allow mothers and infants to remain together— 24 hours a day.

7.1 Do mothers and infants remain together (rooming-in or bedding-in) 24 hours a day, except for periods of up to an hour for hospital procedures or if separation is medically indicated?. . . . . Yes ☐ No ☐

7.2 Does rooming-in start within an hour of a normal birth?. . . . . Yes ☐ No ☐

7.3 Does rooming-in start within an hour when a caesarean mother can respond to her baby? . . . . Yes ☐ No ☐

*Low-cost: below 80% open-market retail cost. Breastmilk substitutes intended for experimental use of "professional evaluation" should also be purchased at 80% or more of retail prices.

STEP 8. Encourage breastfeeding on demand.

8.1 By placing no restrictions on the frequency or length of breastfeeds, do staff show they are aware of the importance of breastfeeding on demand? . . . . Yes ☐ No ☐

8.2 Are mothers advised to breastfeed their babies whenever their babies are hungry and as often as their babies want to breastfeed?. . . . . Yes ☐ No ☐

STEP 9. Give no artificial teats or pacifiers (also called dummies or soothers to breastfeeding infants.

9.1 Are babies who have started to breastfeed cared for without any bottlefeeds?. . . . . Yes ☐ No ☐

9.2 Are babies who have started to breastfeed cared for without using pacifiers?. . . . . .Yes ☐ No ☐

9.3 Do breastfeeding mothers learn that they should not give any bottles or pacifiers to their babies?. . . . . Yes ☐ No ☐

9.4 By accepting no free or low-cost feeding bottles, teats, or pacifiers, do the facility and the health workers demonstrate that these should be avoided?. . . . . Yes ☐ No ☐

STEP 10. Foster the establishment of breastfeeding support and refer mothers to them on discharge from the hospital or clinic.

10.1 Does the hospital give education to key family members so that they can support the breastfeeding mother at home?. . . . . Yes ☐ No ☐

10.2 Are breastfeeding mothers referred to breastfeeding support groups, if any are available?. . . . . Yes ☐ No ☐

10.3 Does the hospital have a system of follow-up support for breastfeeding mothers after they are discharged, such as early postnatal or lactation clinic check-ups, home visits, telephone calls?. . . . . Yes ☐ No ☐

10.4 Does the facility encourage and facilitate the formation of mother-to-mother or healthcare worker-to-mother support groups?. . . . . Yes ☐ No ☐

10.5 Does the facility allow breastfeeding counseling by trained mother-support group counselors in its maternity services?. . . . . Yes ☐ No ☐

Appendix A-19

INFANT BREASTFEEDING ASSESSMENT TOOL (IBFAT)

Infant Breastfeeding Assessment Tool (IBFAT)

Check the score which best describes the baby's feeding behaviours at this feed.

	3	2	1	0
In order to get baby to feed:	Placed the baby on the breast as no effort was needed	Used mild stimulation such as unbundling, patting or burping	Unbundle baby, sat baby back and forward, rub baby's body or limbs vigorously at beginning and during feeding	Could not be aroused
Rooting	Rooted effectively at once	Needed coaxing prompting, or encourgement	Rooted poorly even with coaxing	Did not root
How long from placing baby on breast to latch & suck	0-3 min.	3-10 min.	Over 10 min.	Did not feed
Sucking pattern	Sucked well throughout on one or both breasts	Sucked on & off but needed encouragement	Sucked poorly, weak sucking; sucking efforts for short periods	Did not suck

MOTHER'S EVALUATION

How do you feel about the way the baby fed at this feeding?

3 Very Pleased   2 Pleased   1 Fairly pleased   0 Not pleased

---

IBFAT assigns a score, 0,1, 2, or 3 to five factors. Scores range from 0 to 12. The mother's evaluation score is not calculated in the IBFAT score.

Matthews, MK. (1988). Developing an instrument to assess infant breastfeeding behavior in the early neonatal period. Midwifery 4, 154-65.

* This sheet may be freely copied.

LATCH - Breastfeeding Charting System ©

	0	1	2
L **LATCH**	· Too sleepy or reluctant · No latch achieved	· Repeated attempts · Hold nipple in mouth · Stimulate to suck	· Grasps breast · Tongue down · Lips flanged · Rhythmical sucking
A **AUDIBLE SWALLOWING**	· None	· A few with stimulation	· Spontaneous and Intermittent < 24° · Spontaneous and Frequent
T **TYPE OF NIPPLE**	· Inverted	· Flat	· Everted (after stimulation)
C **COMFORT (Breast/Nipple)**	· Engorged · Cracked, bleeding, lg.blisters or bruises · Severe discomfort	· Filling · Reddened/small blisters or bruises · Mild/moderate discomfort	· Soft · Non-Tender
H **HOLD (Positioning)**	· Full assist (staff holds)	· Minimal assist (i.e., pillows, ↑ HOB) · Teach one side, Mom does other · Staff holds -> Mom takes over	· No assist from staff · Mom able to position/hold baby

Copyright © Nursing Services Division, Sacred Heart General Hospital
From: Jensen, D, Wallace, S., and Kelsay, P. (1994). LATCH: A breastfeeding charting system and documentation tool. JOGNN **23**, 27-32.

*This sheet may be freely copied.

LATCH - Breastfeeding Charting System

Definition of the LATCH Charting System:

1. Each letter of the acronym LATCH denotes an area of breastfeeding assessment.
   L = Latch - how well the baby attaches to the breast.
   A = Audible Swallowing - how frequent swallows are heard.
   T = Type - the type of nipple the mother has after stimulation.
   C = Comfort - how comfortable the mom's breast and nipples feel.
   H = Hold (positioning) - How much help does the mother need in holding/positioning her baby on the breast.
2. A number (0, 1 or 2) is assigned to each letter that is reflective of the degree to which each area of assessment is met. (See below).
3. The numbers are then added up for a total LATCH score. The range is 0 to 10.

Standards of Documentation:

1. On the LATCH grid, enter the time of the breastfeeding and assign a score to each letter based on the assessment done. Total the score and initial. The grid needs to be used for all feedings, observed and reported.
2. Initial box marked "Observed" for an observed assessment.
3. Initial box marked "Reported" for a reported assessment.
4. "Slept" may be used if the baby did not nurse, and no attempt was made to awaken the baby.
5. "R side", "L side", "Both sides", "With shield" may also be used in addition to the LATCH score.
6. Add comments or interventions as needed.
7. When the baby is weighed before and after a feeding, chart breast milk volume in cc's in box marked "Total".

Charting an OBSERVED Breastfeeding:
Observed scoring is assessed as follows:

Latch

2 = All of the following criteria are met:
- Baby's gum line is placed over the mother's lactiferous sinuses 3/4 -1 inch from end of nipple.
- Both lips are flanged outward.
- Jaw movement is visible at ear or temple area.
- Tongue is positioned under the areola.
- Adequate suction is demonstrated by full cheeks, without dimpling.
- Rhythmical sucking occurs with a sustained latch and sucking occurring in bursts of 6-7 compressions every 10 seconds.

1 = The above criteria is only met after repeated attempts and/or the staff must hold the nipple in the mouth and/or stimulate the baby repeatedly to suck.

0 = The baby is too sleepy or reluctant to nurse and no latch is achieved.

Audible Swallowing

2 = Swallowing is heard as resembling a short forceful expiration of air. In the first 24-48 hours, several bursts of sucking may precede the swallowing sound. As milk volume increases (3-4 days after birth), the suck/swallow ratio is 1-2/second.

1 = Swallowing is heard infrequently and usually only with stimulation.

0 = No swallows are heard.

Type

2 = Everted, projects forward after stimulation if necessary.

1 = Flat, does not project forward or minimally.

0 = Inverted, projected inward.

Comfort: Breast

2 = When breasts are physically inspected, they are soft with elastic breast tissue.

1 = When inspected, breasts are filling, becoming fuller and round with decreasing tissue elasticity.

0 = When inspected, breasts are engorged, firm, often tender, with non-elastic breast tissue.

Comfort: Nipple

2 = Mother states nipples are not tender and there are no visible signs of redness, trauma, bruising, blistering, bleeding or cracks.

1 = Mother states there is mild/moderate tenderness. Nipples can be reddened or have small blisters or bruises.

0 = Mother states there is severe discomfort and the nipples are cracked, bleeding, very reddened or have large blisters or areas of bruising.

Hold/Positioning

2 = The mother is able to position the baby at the breast (cradle, football or sidelying) without the assistance of the staff. When observing the positioning, the baby's body should be flexed with no muscular rigidity present. The baby's head should be aligned with the trunk so the head is straight on the breast and not turned laterally or hyperextended. Pillows should be used so the baby's head and body are at breast level. The mother should be supporting her breast with cupped hand.

1 = Assistance is needed by the nursing staff to instruct in positioning or attachment at the first breast and mother attaching baby to the second breast, placing pillows and helping mother to sit up in bed.

0 = Full assistance from the nursing staff to attach the baby, needs to hold the baby in place for the entire feeding.

Charting a REPORTED Breastfeeding:

Reported: A reported LATCH Score can be determined when a feeding was a not observed by asking the mother the following questions:

L **Latch** - How easily did the baby grasp the breast? Did it take several attempts?

A **Audible Swallowing** - Did you hear the baby swallow? How frequent?

T **Type of Nipple** - Do your nipples stand out well? (An assumption can be made here that the mother has fairly everted nipples if the baby is able to grasp the nipples well.)

C **Comfort of Breast/Nipple** - Are your nipples tender? Is your milk beginning to come in?

H **Hold/Positioning** - Would you like help nursing next time? (Most mothers will score a 2 in this category when using reported score, otherwise the nursing staffing would have been assisting and observing the feeding.)

©Nursing Service Division
Sacred Heart Medical Center

CHART TIME AND INITIAL IF ACTIVITY OBSERVATION, OR CARE HAS BEEN GIVEN UNEVENTFULLY.

CROSS OUT ANY CATEGORIES THAT ARE NOT APPLICABLE. SPACE ON BACK IF NEEDED FOR NON-ROUTINE CARE OR TEACHING.

SYSTEMS REVIEW (Initial if asymptomatic Circle & explain if abnormal)

OBSERVATIONS: ADDITIONAL SPACE ON BACK FC DETAILED CHARTING WHERE INDICATED. CROSS O UNUSED LINES AND SIGN ALL ENTRIES.

V.S.: AP T R Ax RESP.						**TIME**	
Physical Care: Bath Cord						CNS	
Feedings Time					Comments/Interventions	Resp.	
L						CV	
A						GI	
T						GU	
C						MS	
H						Integ.	
Total						Mother/Infant Interaction	
Observed/ Reported						I.D. Bands	MD/PNP Exam PKU Circ
Bottle						Teaching	
Elimination: VOID STOOL						2300-0700 Signatures	LPN CNA F

V.S.: AP T R Ax RESP.						**TIME**	
Weight gms. lbs. ozs.						CNS	
Physical Care: Bath Cord							
FeedingsTime					Comments/Interventions	Resp.	
L						CV	
A						GI	
T						GU	
C						MS	
H						Integ.	
Total						Mother/Infant Interaction	
Observed/ Reported						I.D. Bands	MD/PNP Exam PKU Circ
Bottle						Teaching	
Elimination: VOID STOOL						0700-1500 Signatures	LPN CNA F

V.S.: AP T R Ax RESP.						**TIME**	
Physical Care: Bath Cord						CNS	
Feedings Time					Comments/Interventions	Resp.	
L						CV	
A						GI	
T						GU	
C						MS	
H						Integ.	
Total						Mother/Infant Interaction	
Observed/ Reported						I.D. Bands	MD/PNP Exam PKU Circ
Bottle						Teaching	
Elimination: VOID STOOL						1500-2300 Signatures	LPN CNA F

Patient Information

APPROVED ON SIX-MONTH TRIAL AUG. 31, 1991.
CONTACT DIR. OF MEDICAL RECORDS FOR COMMENTS

10000882/12-

Sacred Heart General Hospital

Infant Nursing Care Record

MOTHER-BABY ASSESSMENT (MBA) FORM*

Mother-Baby Assessment Scoring Table Score 0-10

	1	1	Score
Readiness	Baby gives readiness cues: rooting, suckling mouthing	Mother puts baby to breast	
Position	Mother hold baby in good alignment within latch-on range of nipple	Baby roots well at nipple	
Latch-on	Mother assists baby as needed; shows good timing brings baby in close	Baby latches on and sucks well; demonstrates good burst-pause pattern	
Milk Transfer	Mother feels any of the following: thirst, cramps increased lochia; breast ache or tingling, relaxation sleepiness	Baby swallows audibly, spits up milk when burping; milk is observed in baby mouth or dripping from opposite breast	
Outcome	Baby releases breast spontaneously, appears satiated relaxed, falls asleep	Mother's breasts are comfort -able after nursing; no lumps, engorgement, nipple soreness	

From: Mulford, C. (1992). The mother-baby assessment (MBA): An "Apgar Score" for breastfeeding. Jr. Human Lactation **8**,79-82.

* This sheet may be freely copied.